INTERMITTENT FASTING
A COMPLETE GUIDE TO WEIGHT LOSS AND CLEAN EATING

Second Edition

BY NATASHA BROWN

All information is intended only to help you cooperate with your doctor, in your efforts toward desirable weight levels and health. Only your doctor can determine what is right for you. In addition to regular check ups and medical supervision, from your doctor, before starting any other weight loss program, you should consult with your personal physician.

INTERMITTENT FASTING:
How Intermittent Fasting Can Launch You Onto The Road Of Weight Loss, Improved Health, Mental Acuity and Increased Longevity

TABLE OF CONTENTS

Introduction

In the world of health, nutrition and weight loss, intermittent fasting has been getting quite a bit of press in the last few years. What you might not realize is that far from merely being the latest trend and brainchild of some celebrity personal trainer/nutritionist, intermittent fasting has been in existence for thousands of years! I have chosen to write this book for several reasons. First of all, I want to dispel some of the popular myths about intermittent fasting. Second, through the presentation of historical facts and the science behind fasting, I want to advocate for the efficacy of intermittent fasting. Finally, as someone who has incorporated intermittent fasting into their health regime, I want to expose you, the reader, to several variations of intermittent fasting, answer common questions people have about this health practice, offer you practical tips and tricks to get the most out of your intermittent fasting experience, help you avoid fasting mistakes and ultimately, give you the information and advice that will allow you to incorporate this health practice into your health regime as a positive life choice, that will empower you for the rest of your life!

Let's begin with the myth debunking...
- You need to eat often to burn calories. This is just not always true. I will get into the details of how your body processes a meal later in this book, but basically, many

experts consider that you can't fool your body into speeding up its metabolism and burning more calories by eating more frequently.

- When you intermittently fast, your body thinks you're "starving" and shuts down. Again, not true. You can't trick your body into thinking it's starving by skipping meals or fasting for a finite amount of time.
- When you fast, you lose muscle. On the contrary. When you fast, you lose fat and may, over time, actually gain lean muscle.
- You should never skip breakfast. This particular myth may actually have two sources. The people we normally associate with skipping breakfast are often overweight people without a disciplined eating regime intermittent fasting requires a disciplined eating regime. Also, the marketers of breakfast foods; i.e., cereal manufacturers, have a BIG interest in keeping the breakfast myth alive.
- "Eat breakfast like a king, lunch like a queen and dinner like a pauper". We've all heard this one at some point in our dieting lives. The truth is that the time of day you eat something has no effect on how fast or slow you burn the calories. This can be easily proven by studies that have been conducted on people who fast because of

religious reasons, and eat large amounts of food late at night after the sun has set.

- Fasting is just plain BAD for you. I end with this myth, because, ironically, by reading the rest of this book, you will find that not only is fasting NOT bad for your health, but it can profoundly improve your body by increasing insulin sensitivity and decreasing inflammation, improve your mind by boosting levels of beneficial brain hormones and improve your life, affecting genes that control protection against disease as well as longevity.

Intermittent Fasting is not a diet. It is a life choice. Diets ultimately don't work because once you finish the diet, and abandon the strict disciplines of said diet that allowed you to lose weight in the first place, unless you find a solid maintenance plan, you will regain the original weight you lost, and worse, may even add additional pounds. Intermittent Fasting can be used both to lose weight AND maintain weight loss. It is a discipline that will allow you to transition from an overweight state into a healthy weight state and will help you, as long as you choose to follow this discipline, to maintain and prolong a balanced, healthy lifestyle for the rest of your life. Viewed in this light, I believe intermittent fasting has the ability to inspire, motivate and sustain positive, healthful personal growth. Proof of the potential physical, mental and spiritual benefits of intermittent fasting can be found throughout history, in the health regimes of countless elite athletes, living and competing in the present day and innumerable scientific studies being conducted to advance the quality of life for future generations.

If I haven't yet managed to convince you to read further, there is one more reason to consider embracing the lifestyle choice of intermittent fasting. Unlike diets, intermittent fasting doesn't ban certain foods. Sustained positive choice always requires balance. In the case of intermittent fasting, this balance is centered between indulgence and disciplined restraint. There will always be food-centered holidays and celebrations, and with the mindful planning and discipline that intermittent fasting entails, these occasions can be experienced fully without guilt or shame, with the supportive knowledge that tomorrow is truly another day that can balance the excesses of the past with a sensible, healthy, reliable intermittent fasting regime. It is only when you "celebrate" with food every day, that the balance is tipped and weight gain and other systemic health problems are given the opportunity to emerge.

Please note: Everyone's individual health base line is different and may require customized adaptations to a generic lifestyle choice. I urge you to share your plans to add intermittent fasting into your health regime with a medical professional before starting any type of program, to ensure you are proceeding in the most healthful and beneficial way for your individual health concerns.

The History of Fasting

This section has been included to conclusively prove that fasting has been around as long as civilization, and as a matter of fact, arguably even before, as can be witnessed by your pet dog or cat's fasting behavior when they have eaten something that doesn't agree with them or suffered some other illness. For the purposes of this book, I am focusing on the history of fasting as it pertains to religious, spiritual and medical usage.

Let's start with religious fasting. Excepting Zoroastrianism, a religion founded by a Persian prophet that forbids fasting (but does avoid eating meat four days a month!), one can hardly name a religion that does not historically include fasting in its observances in one fashion or another, for a wide spectrum of reasons.

Normally, the go-to source for religious fasting is the period of Ramadan, an approximately month-long period of time observed by Muslims around the world. During this period, eating and drinking is abstained from during daylight hours. The fast is then broken after sunset, usually by a large meal. Fasting is observed during Ramadan as an act of abstinence, as they strive to cleanse both body and soul and increase taqwa, or good deeds.

Muslims have always believed that by reducing overindulgence in food and eating only enough to quell hunger pangs, as well as maintaining normal daily physical activity during Ramadan, they are viscerally reaffirming their religious goals of always striving to attain virtuous behavior, character and habits in thought and deed. Christianity also has a long rich history of fasting, most notably during the Lenten period when fasting is also required by Roman Catholics as an act of abstinence and to represent and reenact the 40 days and nights Jesus spent alone, fasting in the wilderness.

In Judaism, fasting requires complete abstinence from food and drink, including water, and occurs on 6 days of the year, most notably Yom Kippur, which is considered the most important day of the Jewish year. Fasting on Yom Kippur represents atonement and repentance for all one's sins and transgressions from the past year.

Many Buddhist monks and nuns follow Vinaya rules and rarely eat after each day's noon meal. They do not consider this a fast, but more a part of their disciplined regimen, which they believe, helps them in meditation and general good health.

As I mentioned at the beginning of this chapter, there are many lesser known fasting traditions and rituals associated with religion and spirituality around the world. Here is just a sampling of a few of them:

- Eastern Orthodoxy: Fasting is tied to the principle between the body (Soma) and the soul (Pnevma). Orthodox Christians regard body and soul as a single unity and believe that what happens to one has an effect on the other (known as the Psychosomatic Union). Fasting takes up much of the

Eastern Orthodox calendar and is not enacted to suffer, but rather to guard against gluttony as well as negative thoughts, words and deeds. The fasting is always accompanied by prayer and almsgiving, or donations to charity or individuals in need.

- Church of the East: All Christians of Syriac traditions have practiced a pre-Lenten fasting event called the Nineveh Fast since the 6th century! During that time, a plague afflicted this region, which we now know as modern-day Iraq. Out of fear and desperation the people ran to their Bishop for a solution. The Bishop referred to scripture and ordered a three-day fast to ask God for forgiveness, based upon the story of Jonah in the Old Testament. Legend has it that after the three days the plague disappeared.

- Mormons: Members of the Mormon Church are encouraged to fast the first Sunday of each month. During these "Fast Sundays" they skip two meals for a total of 24 hours. Any money they save by not purchasing or preparing these two meals is donated to the church, which, in turn uses the money to help the needy.

- Hinduism: Fasting takes on many forms and variations in the Hindu religion, based on personal beliefs and local custom. Certain days of the week are designated for one's personal creed as well as favorite deities. Thursdays, for example, are a common fasting day for Hindus of northern India, who wear yellow clothing and worship Vrhaspati Mahadeva or Guru.

- Yoga: Practitioners of the yoga principle believe a fast should be maintained on the Full Moon day of each month, and to spend the entire day with a positive spiritual attitude
- Taoism: Fasting practices originated as a Daoist technique for becoming immortal and later became a traditional Chinese medical cure for Sanshi, or the "Three corpses", life-shortening spirits thought to reside in the human body.
- Sikhism: Sikhs only believe in fasting for medical reasons and when fasting for health are encouraged to remember to act with honesty, sincerity and to control desires.

Interestingly, no matter the form, intensity, length or reasoning for fasting in these religions and spiritual groups, all recommend cautions to individuals who are in some way not capable physically of the rigors of abstaining from nutrition. These include: children, the elderly, those who are medically fragile, pregnant, nursing or menstruating women. I think it is wise to take a page from these sometimes ancient fasting rules and exceptions, and always seek medical treatment before beginning any form of intermittent fasting.

The medical history of fasting is as fascinating and diverse in its own right. Pythagoras (580-500 BC), the famous Greek mathematician and philosopher, purposely fasted for 40-day periods, believing that it increased mental acuity and creativity. He demanded the same strict fasting periods from his disciples and followers. Hippocrates (460-357BC) the "father of medicine" and inspiration of the Hippocratic oath, which must be sworn by all medical doctors to this day was an advocate of moderation and treatment through fasting, believing "when a patient is fed too richly, the disease is fed as well. Remember – any excess is against nature." Fasting as a medical treatment continued through the middle Ages and had resurgence during the Renaissance. Luigi di Cornaro, a Venetian aristocrat, credited fasting with saving his life, writing "A Treatise on temperate living" in tribute to its life changing benefits. German physician and chemist Friedrich Hoffmann (1660-1742) used limotherapy, or the voluntary temporary abstention of food to treat many ailments, including plethora, arthritis, apoplexy, skin disease and cataracts. His first rule of treatment: "For each disease, for the patient it is the best not to eat anything." Famous patriot, inventor and founding father of America, Benjamin Franklin was a fierce advocate of fasting, claiming

"The best of all medicines is rest and fasting". In 1877, Dr. Edward Dewey, an American physician, pioneered the implementation of long term fasting for its curative powers. He believed that if a patient presented symptoms including loss of appetite and a coated tongue, s/he should fast until these symptoms disappeared.

Therapeutic fasting became more and more popular through end of the 19th century and continued on into the early 20th century in Europe, and fasting resorts opened to treat patients. American naturopath, Herbert McGolfin Shelton, who supervised the fasts of over 40,000 clients, lived for 100 years and was nominated by the American Vegetarian Party to run for President in 1956, wrote, "Fasting must be recognized as a fundamental and radical process that is older than any other mode of caring for the sick organism, for it is employed on the plane of instinct..." During this century, fasting was used to treat a range of health ailments including heart disease, high blood pressure, obesity, digestive problems, allergies and headaches.

To this day in Germany, fasting is part of "nuturheilkunde" – natural health practice, and has been integrated into medical practice to the point that patients can be referred for a fast by their doctors.

The practice of intermittent fasting has brought this ageless practice full circle, proving the axiom, "everything old is new again!" Intermittent fasting seems to have entered the diet and health scene around the turn of the new millennium and, not surprisingly, during the early days of the Internet. Books like "The Warrior Diet" by Ori Hofmekler and "Eat Stop Eat." By Brad Pilon, pioneered the principles of intermittent fasting and then in 2007, Martin Berkhan burst onto the Internet scene with "Lean Gains", bringing awareness of intermittent fasting to mainstream audiences and becoming the face of the movement. Since then, countless health, nutrition and fitness communities including Paleo and CrossFit have adapted intermittent fasting to their own regimes.

Whether you ultimately choose to follow one of the many well-established intermittent fasting programs or customize intermittent fasting to your individual needs, it's reassuring to know that this is not just the latest dieting fad or trend. It is a lifestyle choice with deep roots in the history of humankind.

In the next chapter, I will explain exactly what happens when your body is in a fasted state, rather than a fed state, as well as how fasting affects how we burn and store calories and how we detoxify.

The Science Behind Intermittent Fasting

One mission I had when I decided to write this book was to figure out how to explain what actually happens IN your body when you intermittently fast. I personally don't support it when writers either patronizingly gloss over HOW intermittent fasting works, as if it was just too complicated for mere mortals to understand, or write exclusively in scientific terms and jargon, losing the reader who isn't incapable of understanding, but simply doesn't understand the language! Also, like many of you, I'm just a little too practical to simply accept someone promising me that if I fast intermittently, all sorts of magical things will happen to me. So...let's keep it simple but straightforward!

When it comes to eating and digesting food our bodies are in one of two states:

- The FED State – When we are in the active process of eating or within a few hours of eating.
- The FASTING State – When we haven't eaten for 6 hours or more.

I think it's interesting to note, that unless you get up in the middle of the night for a snack, pretty much everyone experiences being in a fasting state every night; a.k.a, sleep!

If we spend our days eating frequently, or at least at intervals of less than 6 hours, we stay in some area of the FED state at all times. That means we are constantly in the process of digestion and elimination.

If we begin to incorporate intermittent fasting into our eating regime, we begin to SCHEDULE periods of time of longer than 6 hours (when we aren't asleep) and allow our bodies the opportunity to experience entering the FASTING state more frequently.

What happens when our bodies are in the FASTING State?

- We burn through our normal energy stores of sugar, or GLUCOSE
- We find alternate sources of energy to burn in our body, including old protein, consisting of connective tissue, skin, old cells and other deitrus, which needs to be eliminated as well as...FAT!

If we were to stop right here, I think it's pretty obvious we could easily conclude that fasting helps our bodies not only burn energy sources more efficiently, but also repurposes fat and other undesirable elements in our body as alternative energy sources. In this way, not only are we thoroughly using up ALL energy resources, good and bad, but also, we are detoxing our bodies of old, used up material at the same time!

Here are a few more things that happen when our bodies are in a FASTING State:

- Leptin and Ghrelin Levels– Leptin and Ghrelin are basically the "appetite" hormones. Leptin tells your body to store fat and sends you hunger signals. Ghrelin tells your brain that your body is hungry. When your body is in a FASTING State it allows the panic buttons of Leptin and Ghrelin to be RESET! Thus, these two alarmist hormones settle down and stop being the "little boys who cried HUNGRY" all the time.

- Autophagy – This is a fancy word for the deep-cleaning process that our miraculous bodies attempt to do on top of everything else 24/7. Eating and Digestion get in the way of this process. However, when a body is in FASTING State, the digestive system gets a well-deserved break and clears the path for Autophagy to occur. Between our fasting bodies burning up fat stores and old used up bodily materials and focused periods of Autophagy, fasting enables our bodies to experience a good old-fashioned Autumn Leaf Fire and a thorough Spring Cleaning in one fell swoop!

These are just a few of the endlessly fascinating things that happen in our bodies when they are experiencing a FASTING State. If you, like me are a lifelong student -- the continued study of intermittent fasting will open up the door to endless learning opportunities. The more we understand how our bodies operate, as well as how best to maintain them, the more they will thank and reward us throughout our lifetime.

The Benefits of Intermittent Fasting

I think already, it is becoming quite obvious that Intermittent Fasting can be an effective and beneficial lifestyle choice for people looking to recover and/or maintain their health. While I tried to focus only on the history and science of fasting in the first two chapters, it became increasingly difficult to explore these two elements of intermittent fasting without touting at least a few of the benefits – as a form of spiritual communication, as an alternative health therapy throughout history and as a caloric regulator and physiological detoxifier.

In this chapter, I want to expand upon the list of the potential benefits of intermittent fasting and include as many lenses as possible through which to view the opportunities and rewards of this popular and effective health and wellness regime.

Physical Benefits

- Weight loss – intermittent fasting, when paired with clean, organic nutritious food eaten in moderation and the added bonus of physical activity, can result in steady, consistent weight loss that stays off!

- Targeted Belly Fat Loss – this harmful abdominal cavity fat can deposit around your internal organs and release proteins and hormones, which causes inflammation and may affect how well you break down sugars and fats. Intermittent fasting is the ideal solution for this stubborn weight gain,

when paired with sugar reduction, increased healthy fats, sleep and stress reduction.
- Maintenance and potential gain of lean muscle mass – Many weight trainers and other elite athletes swear by intermittent fasting when training to help them maintain lean muscle mass and decrease total body fat.

Mental Benefits

- Improved metabolism, which is beneficial to Brain Health, Metabolism is the name for the crucial chemical reactions that happen in your cells. We talk about having a fast or slow metabolism all the time, without really understanding how vital it is to conversion of food to fuel, composing the building blocks for proteins and carbohydrates and the elimination of cellular waste.
- Improved Ketone production. Ketone is a chemical that protects the brain when there is a decrease of available glucose.
- May reduce symptoms of depression by regulating insulin and blood sugar levels.
- Enhances performance on memory tests in the elderly
- May play preventative role in those suffering from anxiety through regulation

of glucose and decreased oxidative stress. Oxidative stress happens when the body can't detox the harmful effects of free radicals (uncharged molecules) fast enough.

Systemic Benefits

- Cellular Repair – through autophagy, which is given more focus in a FASTING State.
- Hormonal Rebalancing – Insulin Levels and Insulin Resistance; Leptin; Ghrelin Also, Human Growth Hormone increases and facilitates fat burning and muscle gain
- Gene protection – Related to longevity and protection against diseases, including promising research on cancer
- Reduces Oxidative stress, damage and inflammation in the body

Quality of Life Benefits

- May improve sleep patterns – If your intermittent fasting schedule includes eating a meal 3 to 4 hours before sleeping, and includes carbohydrates, your sleep quality and quantity could improve due to increased production of serotonin, a chemical in the body that helps regulate cyclic body processes, such as the sleep cycle, as well as contributing to feelings of happiness and wellbeing.

- Increased stamina – Athletes who exercise on an empty stomach have experienced more energy and stamina. It is believed that the combination of fasting and exercising triggers internal catalysts that force the breakdown of sugars and fat into energy, without sacrificing muscle mass.

Behavioral Benefits

- Improves appetite control – Intermittent Fasting allows you to discern between mental and physical hunger
- Helps with food cravings – As your Leptin and Ghrelin levels reset to your intermittent fasting schedule, old triggers to eat certain foods at certain times will be erased. Also, intermittent fasting doesn't ban certain foods; only the time period in which you can consume them!
- Develops an appreciation for high quality food—when you learn to eat within a certain time frame, and fast through another, you learn to appreciate the gift of eating good quality food. You may notice that you savor food more, eating it more slowly, and that you have a much keener sense of when you are becoming full. You will also discover certain, high quality food

sources such as whey protein, green vegetables and berries are ingested and incorporated faster into your system, due to their nutritionally dense makeup.

Fiscal and Time-Saving Benefits

- Save money – Depending on your intermittent fasting schedule, you could end up skipping 7 meals or more a week. As long as you don't add the caloric totals of these meals to the meals you DO consume during intermittent fasting, you are basically cutting at least a day's worth of food out of your budget. Take a page from the Mormon faith and add up how much money you save by not purchasing and preparing these meals. Whether you pay that savings forward or save it for a rainy day is up to you!
- Save time – This particular benefit personally resonates with me. As a former dieter, I can say with the voice of an expert, that many of the miracle diets and fads I tried, in my quest to lose weight, not only included lots of really expensive ingredients in little quantities that resulted in even more waste, but the elaborate preparation required of these meals, took hours away from my life that I would never

get back. When you choose to fast intermittently, you automatically save a certain percentage of weekly food prep basically because you SKIP the entire process. It's up to you how plain or fancy your remaining meals are. The important thing is to eat a balanced, clean, organic nutritious menu of food. And if you overindulge a day or two on vacation? Tomorrow is truly another day.

Personal Growth Benefits

- Taking a on a physical and mental challenge and being rewarded with the ability to balance health and nutritional needs.
- Acquiring a great tool for strength training or other athletic challenges.
- Experiencing consistent balanced control over important life choices.
- Gaining the flexibility and freedom to choose when you eat socially with friends and family, and when you take a planned break.
- Experiencing Mind/Body connection in a visceral manner that regulates when, why and how you eat.
- Learning how to be mindful when eating
- Experiencing delayed gratification rather than immediate gratification
- Developing resilience in a controlled setting

- Learning how to respect boundaries and how to be nutritionally creative within them

As I hope you can see by the diverse spectrum of benefits I've included above, I personally believe that the practice of Intermittent Fasting offers you much, much more than a diet. As I've stated before, it's an important, valuable life choice – the rewards that will be gained from incorporating it into your health regime can easily be scaffolded into many other parts of your life. I am a big advocate of connecting mind, body and spirit into a cohesive, healthy, balanced whole, transforming us all into empowered individuals; ready to take on all the opportunities this world has to offer!

Three Major Types of Intermittent Fasting

Intermittent Fasting, as we know it today, has been in existence roughly since the turn of the millennium. In the past seventeen years, it has gained more and more traction, as more research is conducted, more health, nutrition and athletic groups have incorporated it into their programs and more and more people have adopted it as a viable, sustainable life choice. When you think about it, almost two decades is an impressive run for something that was initially dismissed by many as an unhealthy fad! There are probably as many variations of intermittent fasting on the market today as there are health and wellness sites, so in order to expose you to as wide a selection of available plans within the confines of this book, I have chosen to focus on three major types: Whole Day Fasting (WDF); 5:2 Intermittent Fasting; and Timed Restricted Fasting (TRF).

Whole Day Fasting (WDF)

Whole Day Fasting was developed and made popular by Brad Pilon, who wrote the book, *Eat Stop Eat*. The basic concept of this intermittent fasting plan is to fast for 24 hours once or twice a week. During the fasting period, no food is consumed but calorie-free beverages are freely permitted (and encouraged). A typical fast day might start after your evening meal, at 7 pm on a Tuesday. You then would fast from all food until 7 pm on Wednesday, at which time you would go back to normal eating. For the next couple of days, you would eat normally (about 2000 calories for women; 2500 for men) and then you would have another 24 hour fast and repeat the schedule. The main rule would be NEVER to fast for two days in a row, or fast more than two times in one week. Maintenance of whole day fasting like this would result in cutting 2/7 of your normal weekly food consumption.

Optimally, your caloric goal on fast days would be as little as possible, drinking tea, coffee, plain or sparkling water and other zero-calorie beverages. The key to non-fasting days would be moderation and balance, as overeating on these days could start to undo what you accomplished during the fast. This is especially important if you are intermittently fasting with the primary goal of losing weight. However, you do not have to avoid any specific foods, although lots of fruits, vegetables and spices are recommended.

Pilon specifically developed this particular intermittent fasting plan as part of a fitness regime that included resistance and weight training to maintain and build lean muscle, rather than cardio-based routines, which might be too taxing, especially on fasting days. The recommended training schedule would be 3 to 4 times a week.

5:2 Intermittent Fasting

5:2 fasting, also known as The Fast Diet, was popularized by Michael Mosley, a British doctor. Like Whole Day Fasting, participants eat normally 5 days of the week, but instead of a complete fast on the other 2 days, restrict calories to 500-600 a day. This eating pattern depends more on timing than food choice and only requires counting calories two days a week, but is obviously, not as restrictive as the 24 hour fasting periods of Whole Day Fasting. Many who choose this form of intermittent fasting, designate Mondays and Thursdays as the two days they reduce caloric intake to between 500 (for women) and 600 (for men) calories. Whichever days you choose, the one rule is to have at least ONE non-fasting day between the two fasting days.

Mosely recommends eating 3 small or 2 slightly bigger meals a day on the 2 fasting days, and to focus on high fiber, high protein foods that will help you feel full without extra calorie consumption. Your total caloric consumption on fast days should equal 25% of your normal daily food consumption. Therefore, in one week you would theoretically be cutting out 75% of your calories on 2 out of 7 days, IF you don't go over 2000 (women) or 2400 (men) calories a day on the remaining 5 days.

The 5:2 plan also advocates exercise, and basically says, with medical clearance, that after the initial transition weeks, ANY exercise regime that is normally followed can be continued through fast days, although again, intense cardio is not specifically advocated.

The 5:2 plan also takes BMI (Body Mass Index), BMR (Basal Metabolic Rate) and TDEE (Total Daily Energy Expenditure) into account. BMI calculates how much body fat you have, in proportion to your height and weight. BMI measures the amount of calories you would burn if you just sat and did nothing for a 24-hour period. TDEE equals the number of calories you consume in a day when your BMR is scaled to a level of activity. In other words, how many calories a day you need to maintain your current weight, and depending upon how active you are, how many calories a day you should consume on the 5 days you aren't fasting.

Although this gets a bit technical and may seem to fly in the face of the principle that intermittent fasting is great because you don't need to worry about what you eat on non-fasting days, it's really just a more complicated way to remember moderation, especially if your goal is to lose weight.

Timed Restricted Fasting (TRF)

Time Restricted Fasting also known as Leangains, was developed and popularized by Martin Berkhan, a professional fitness writer and consultant, who revolutionized the fitness scene when he proposed that intermittent fasting was better for athletes in training (specifically body builders) than eating small meals every 2 to 3 hours. The basic concept of Timed Restricted Fasting is to fast for 16 hours a day and then eat in the remaining 8-hour window of time. There are no food restrictions during the 8-hour feeding period, as long as you meet your daily caloric and macronutrient target. What are macronutrients? Macronutrients (or macros) are a fancy term for the types of food needed by a living organism. For humans this means carbohydrates, fats and proteins, which are the three basic components of every diet! Getting the proportions of these three nutrients right makes a big difference, when trying to maintain or lose weight. Some people claim that counting macros is much more effective than counting calories when controlling weight. For the purposes of understanding macros to calories the following explains what each macro counts as, in caloric terms:

- Protein – equal to 4 calories per gram
- Carbohydrates –equal to 4 calories per gram
- Fats – equal to 9 calories per gram

Once you have this formula down, you can determine your personal macronutrient targets. A common split is 40/40/20. In other words, 40% of your calories should be spent on protein, 40% on carbohydrates and 20% on fats. Again, compared to the simplicity of Whole Day Fasting, all of this may seem complicated and defeat the purpose of intermittent fasting, but it really comes down to your personal goals and what level of nutrition and fitness comprehension resonates with you. It can be as simple as moderation or as complex as formulating your daily macronutrient needs – and it means the same thing!

Time Restricted Fasting was specifically designed to be used by body builders who were basically tired of eating constantly like frenzied birds; feeling "half-starved" all of the time and wanted to be able to eat large meals some of the time with relative freedom. It was also designed as a response to athletes who were tired of having to miss many social events, as the timing and food-themed tones of most of them didn't fit into their 2-3 hour mini-meal schedule.

It goes without saying that Time Restricted Fasting advocates for the addition of physical activity, as intense training and intermittent fasting go hand in hand in this particular version. Again, cardio activities take a back seat to resistance and weight training in this scenario.

The three types of Intermittent Fasting I have chosen to highlight in this section are currently among the most popular and trending today, but are certainly NOT the only ways in which you can experience intermittent fasting. Other variations include: *The Warrior Diet*, a 20-hour fasting sequence with one meal a day, written by Ori Hofmekler, *The UpDayDownDay Diet*, written by Dr. James Johnson, which uses an alternative day intermittent fasting approach and focuses on targeting what he refers to as the "skinny" gene, and *Fat Loss Forever*, a hybrid of *Eat Stop Eat*, *Warrior Diet* and *Leangains*, that features a cheat day followed by a 36 hour fast, started by John Romaniello and Dan Go.

Alternatively, once you have a basic understanding of the basic principles of intermittent fasting and have figured out your own goals, there is no reason why you can't pick up your favorite "best practices" from these variations, and devise a customized intermittent fasting program that meets your own needs! I've written the following chapters of this book with the intention of helping you implement the tools of intermittent fasting into your daily life, whether your goals include weight loss, weight maintenance, nutritional improvement and consistency, physical training goals, increased stamina and endurance, appetite control or any of the other numerous nutrition/health and wellness issues that may be interfering with the balance of your daily life. Let's get started!

Intermittent Fasting For Weight Loss And The "Magic Bullet" Of Exercise

If one of your health goals for using intermittent fasting is weight loss, it's important to establish some base lines before starting your journey. First of all, you need to figure out how many calories you need in order to facilitate a healthy weight loss, keeping in mind, that the addition of ANY kind of intermittent fasting practice will automatically eliminate a percentage of calories per time period fasted X how many meals you skip. As I mentioned earlier, then recommended daily calorie intake for maintaining healthy body weight is 2000 for women and 2500 for men. It is also commonly accepted that cutting back 500 calories a day, to 1500 for women and 2000 for men, will optimize weight loss of up to one pound per week.

However, this is only a standard. Everyone is different, and medical needs, stage of life needs, activity levels, etc. should always be factored in. Medical clearance for any sort of weight reduction is recommended, should be sought out as an important source of advice and/or feedback during the weight loss process.

Please don't be disappointed that I am talking about calories and restriction. I know you've probably been excited about intermittent fasting because one if it's most attractive selling points is the "eat all you want" aspect on non-fasting days. If you don't want to lose more than a couple of pounds or are looking to accomplish other health/nutrition goals, this benefit holds fast, albeit, perhaps it should be edited to read "Eat all the clean organic, nutrient dense food you want", or "eat all the macronutrients that will contribute to your lean muscle mass". OKAY... maybe these variations don't exactly say, "Gorge to your heart's content", but compared to many calorie restrictive diets.... It's a good thing!

And speaking of calorie restrictive DIETS...don't you think using the tool of intermittent periods of fasting, interspersed with "normal" periods of moderation sound a heck of a lot better than eating cabbage soup three times a day or prepping 6 mini meals every night before you head to bed? I thought so! Also, when I think of intermittent fasting I think of endless opportunities to get the whole weight loss battle right – if, God forbid, you have an occasional overindulgent non-fasting day all you need to do to reset is go to sleep, unrepentant because tomorrow or the next day offers the opportunity to redeem yourself with a period of fasting. Try that in week two or three of some draconian food-deprived diet and chances are you'll be slipping off that wagon faster than that piece of cake you devoured at your friend's birthday party!

But I digress...If you aren't satisfied with a minimum standard of how many calories you should be consuming per day, including intermittent fasting there is a formula to customize this number for your personal needs. Borrowing from 5:2 intermittent fasting and The Fast Diet, here's how to figure out your TDEE (Total Daily Energy Expenditure):

Note: This formula uses the metric system. 1 kg = 2.2 pounds; 1 inch = 2.54 cm

FIRST: Calculate your BMR (Basal Metabolic Rate)

Women: BMR = 655 + (9.6 X weight in kg) + (1.8 X height in cm) – (4.7 x age in years)

Men: BMR = 66 + (13.7 X weight in kg) + (5 X height in cm) – (6.8 X age in years)
Multiply the number in parenthesis first, then you can add and subtract

EX: Female
Age 55 years
Weight: 197 lbs. (89.54 kg)
Height: 5' 4" (162.56 cm)
655 + (9.6 X433.4 kg) + (1.8 X 162.56 cm) – (4.7 X 55) = 1,549 calories/day (rounded up)

SECOND: Calculate TDEE
TDEE = BMR X Activity Factor

Activity Factor:
Sedentary (little or no exercise) = 1.2

Lightly Active (light exercise 1-3 days/week) = 1.375

Moderately Active (exercise 3-5 days/week) = 1.55

Heavy Exercise (exercise 6-7 days/week) = 1.725

Very Heavy Exercise (physical labor; training 2X/day) = 1.9

EX: 1,549 calories X 1.375 (lightly active) = 2,129 calories a day needed to maintain current weight
In order for this woman to lose approximately 1 pound per week she would need to cut her daily calorie count by 500 calories, adjusting her TDEE to 1,629 calories a day.

WHEWWW! That wasn't easy! The good news is there are calculators and apps that will do all this work for you if math isn't among your strong suits. However, I always think it's worthwhile to understand how a rate is figured out and the bonus is the one thing that becomes abundantly clear when working out your TDEE is what a powerful tool physical activity can be in your weight loss journey.
How truthful were you when it came to figuring out your Activity Factor? Don't feel bad – most people overestimate how active they are. Were you surprised at how much you needed to move to be considered moderately active? The good news is physical activity; ANY physical activity can be added to your health regime, AT YOUR COMFORT LEVEL. I'm afraid we've all become accustomed to watching extreme weight loss reality shows and falling for the belief that in order to make a difference in weight loss, we need to immediately jump into the fray, overworking ourselves into a

dangerous, sweaty, sobbing mess in order to feel the burn.

FAIL! This is an extremely dangerous way to introduce exercise into your life and the chance of injury or emotional trauma is more than likely to ensure you will think 10 times before attempting to exercise again. Work out in this fashion and you will literally end up THE BIGGEST LOSER.

Instead, I offer you various physical activity options to try out at any level of the activity factor. Please read the following from beginning to end to see the possibilities and opportunities that await a human being currently at any level of fitness:

- Physical Activity Options for the Sedentary: Gentle yoga; chair yoga; walking with a friend; mall walking; tai chi; social dancing, i.e., folk, line, square; walking in a pool; gentle aqua aerobics; lawn games like croquet or bocce; light gardening or yard work. The key is to go at your own pace, stop whenever you need to and ignore people who try to push you beyond your limits. It's a lifelong process – not a race!

- Physical Activity for the Lightly Active: Start taking the stairs more often; park farther from your destination and walk the rest of the way; spring clean once a month; buy a pedometer or Fitbit and start keeping track of your steps; play with your kids or grandkids; go on family walks after dinner.

The key is to begin incorporating physical activity into your daily routine, while keeping up with the fun stuff you started when you were sedentary!

- Physical Activity for the Moderately Active: On days you don't have planned or scheduled physical activities, you should try to aim for 60 minutes of Lifestyle activity which could include house and garden work; biking or hiking with friends and family, swimming in your home pool or going to a lake or ocean beach for the afternoon and spending time swimming organized sports such as work softball or pickup basketball teams; volunteer physical labor for church or community as well as formal gym and swim classes; or scheduled jogging or biking sessions. The key at this point is to celebrate how far you've come from the couch and TV by honing your level of physical fitness in work and play.

- Physical Activity for the Heavy Exerciser: Challenge yourself with CrossFit; competitive sports such as tennis, swimming or ballroom dancing; mountain climbing and biking, cross country ski, long-distance hiking; train for and compete in marathons, and triathlons; cross-country biking vacations and races. Take the skills you've mastered in the gym and implement them in real-life activities. The key at this point is to discover and challenge your fitness at every opportunity. Learn new skills to keep the mind-body connection strong and keep advancing your personal best.

- Physical Activity for the Very Heavy Exerciser: Ironman events; elite tests of endurance such as Tough Guy UK; epic adventure races like Raid Gauloises or the Barkley 100 Trail Race; REI's Mount Kilimanjaro Climb; or elite mud runs like The Spartan Beast, which runs in various cities and dates. Remove any remaining limits and pit your skills against the best in the world! There's always room to grow and physically challenge yourself! Check out these events and more on the Internet. The World is your oyster!

The point of this is – that basically once you begin adding physical activity to your routine, there is literally no end point. Physical fitness at any age, level, ability or disability, knows no limit and is only made more achievable and exciting by the personal boundaries that we choose or that have been thrust upon us! Beginning a program of intermittent fasting is the perfect opportunity to discover the joys of physical fitness, while reaping the calorie burning, body freeing, flexibility and agility benefits that learning to move your body will offer you.

Twenty Questions About Intermittent Fasting!

The aim of this section is to answer any and all questions you might have at this point about intermittent fasting. I've tried to address questions related to fasting for weight loss as well as for people who are looking to maintain and/or otherwise amp up their health and wellness regime. If you have questions I didn't address, please send them in! I love getting feedback from my readers and using it to improve the books I write!

Which type of intermittent fasting should I choose to follow and why?

Many of the reasons for choosing one type of intermittent fasting over another will depend on personal preference, lifestyle as well as short and long-term goals. What I can do for you is list some advantages of each of the 3 types I described earlier in this book.

Whole Day Fasting

- o 1 to 2 days of fasting and 5 days of feeding give you greater flexibility when it comes to eating socially, or at home with family.
- o Works for those who resonate with "all or nothing" mentality
- o Fits in well with vacation and/or holiday plans

o Allows for longer "recovery" time between fasting
o Allows you to "get it all over with" in only 48 hours

5:2 Intermittent Fasting

o The 2 minimal calorie days, still allow you to eat something
o Feels less restrictive than Whole Day Fasting
o Allows you to eat a bit after training session, even on "fast" days
o Appeals to people who have issues about not eating at all for 24 hours
o Might be a great way to introduce yourself or transition into intermittent fasting

Time Restricted Fasting

o More attractive to people who resonate with a more consistent routine
o The ability to fast and eat in one 24-hour period
o The philosophy that every day is a brand-new opportunity to improve
o Less chance of overindulging during feeding periods
o Creates more structured boundaries

Please also remember, that there are many more

types, hybrids and versions of intermittent fasting available to choose from. The most important takeaway is that you find a plan that resonates with you! And if you can't find exactly the right fit for your needs, there's no reason you can't design your own plan. Finally, keeping in mind that ideally, intermittent fasting is a life-long choice, don't limit yourself to one way of fasting. Life changes, and when it does, it's important to be able to flex to new challenges. Fortunately, for us, there are a variety of ways to accomplish intermittent fasting!

How and what should I eat during feeding periods?

The short answer is: Any way and anything you want! The long answer needs to reflect what your nutrition goals are. If you are intermittently fasting to lose weight, you need to eat in moderation and make sure you don't "make up for lost time" in terms of the meals you skipped while fasting. No matter what type of fasting program you are following, it's important to know how many calories you should be aiming for a day, i.e., your TDEE minus 500 calories a day or more, depending on how much weight you would like to lose a week. But remember – if you are fasting, that 500 calories probably has already been saved! Isn't that great news!

If you are practicing intermittent fasting because you are a weight trainer and are sick of eating like a bird every 2 or 3 hours, then your feeding goals are going to be much different. You will need to make sure that you eat everything you missed during the fasting period, during the window of feeding time. Also, what you eat, i.e., how much protein vs how many carbs, will be important to continue to support your training. If you are training for a specific event such as a marathon or triathlon, you may need to up certain food groups, in preparation for the big day.

If you have decided to practice intermittent fasting in order to experience the many health and wellness benefits I listed previously, but you are satisfied with your current weight, you will need to be mindful that you are eating enough to satisfy your TDEE and that those food sources are as nutrient-dense, clean and organic as possible.

Choosing an intermittent fasting lifestyle can mean that an occasional indulgence will be balanced out by the majority of your healthy food choices. It really shouldn't mean that you fast intermittently so that you can binge on junk food and processed, GMO laden prepared foods. Intermittent Fasting is not a giant filter, magically cleansing you of your toxic food choices. It is a lifestyle that allows you to easily balance eating to live and living to eat.

I'm concerned.... Won't this mess up my circadian rhythms?

First of all, let's explain what circadian rhythms are! Basically, your circadian rhythm is your 24-hour internal clock that runs in the background of your consciousness and cycles your body between periods of sleep and wake. It's also known as your sleep/wake cycle. Typically, most adults experience the most profound dip in energy twice in a 24-hour cycle: once somewhere between 2 and 4 am, and once between 1 and 3 pm. These times can shift if you tend to be more nocturnal or a "morning" person. When you experience consistent, quality sleep you won't be as aware of these 2 cyclical decreases in energy.

If you are sleep deprived, you will. The lightness or darkness of your environment can trigger your circadian rhythms, as darkness cues your eyes to tell your brain that it's time to feel tired. Your brain then sends a signal to your body to release the hormone melatonin, which makes you physically tired. So, night and day as well as consistent sleep periods pretty much regulate your circadian rhythms.

Disruptions such as daylight savings time, travelling to another time zone, or watching late night TV can disrupt your circadian rhythms and you will pay for it the next day. Can intermittent fasting also disrupt circadian rhythms? The answer is interesting – it depends! The interesting part is that it is NOT because many intermittent fasting programs skip breakfast (although, as we have discussed several times, intermittent fasting and feeding times can be adjusted to personal preference). In actuality, our hunger is naturally at our lowest point upon waking, increases during the day, and peaks around 7 to 8 at night.

We in western civilization tend eat dinner around this time period because it conveniently coincides from when we get home from work and school commitments and reconvene as a family. Also, our internal levels of insulin are maximally stimulated at this time so eating dinner on the late side starts to feel like the perfect storm. When viewed in this light, no matter how you are eating (intermittently or at will) or what you are eating, doesn't matter as much as when you are eating. Perhaps, if instead we all took a page from the Mediterraneans, who eat their largest meal in the early afternoon, and then siesta it off with an afternoon nap, before returning to work and eating a light meal, later in the evening, we'd all benefit from our hormonal and circadian cycles working in perfect harmony! So bottom line: Intermittent fasting doesn't need to interrupt your circadian rhythm but waiting until 9 o'clock at night to catch up on the bulk of your eating could.

I think I need to take a break on weekends. Can I still do intermittent fasting?

If you choose to follow a daily intermittent fasting plan such as time restricted fasting, the answer is, sadly no – you would have to break the daily pattern to take a break on weekends. If, however you follow an intermittent fasting plan such as whole day intermittent fasting or 5: 2 intermittent fasting the answer to this question is a resounding YES!

In fact, as I believe I mentioned earlier, the recommended days for 5:2 fasting are Mondays and Thursdays, which when you think about it, couldn't work out better for taking the weekend off and indulging just a bit. Your fasting days basically "sandwich" (sorry about the pun!) the weekend, allowing you to eat much more freely, knowing you've just ended a fast and will enter another after the hopefully, minor excesses of the weekend!

I'm really concerned about losing muscle mass. How can I prevent this from happening while training and fasting intermittently?

As I've mentioned before, one of the benefits of using Intermittent Fasting methods while training or working out, is that you tend to lose FAT while maintaining lean muscle mass. But there are additional techniques you can employ to ensure that you will maintain, and if you choose, even gain lean muscle mass while intermittently fasting. Calorie and carbohydrate cycling are both great tools to add to your nutritional program. Cycle calories by eating more on the days you work out and less on your training days. In other words, add or decrease food intake during your feeding times, to coincide with training or rest days. This results in more energy to burn into muscle on training days and fewer calories to burn fat on your resting days.

If you follow this pattern consistently, you should end up having done both in one week. Carbohydrate cycle by increasing carb consumption on training days and decreasing carbs on resting days. The principle works the same way as caloric cycling. Finally, eat high protein all the time and decrease fat intake to moderate or low on resting days.

I'm not fasting to lose weight... How do I manage to eat enough food during my feeding window?

Okay, people who need to lose a few pounds – stop groaning and throwing things! This is just as much of a concern for people as counting calories is for others. When people incorporate intermittent fasting into their training schedule as an alternative to eating every two or three hours throughout the day, they gain time to eat socially with family and friends as well to eat normal sized plates of food, but there is also a transition challenge of eating enough calories when weight loss isn't a goal. Perhaps the easy answer would be to enjoy all that fattening ice-cream, cake and alcohol that most people can't – but we're talking about people who take their health and nutritional needs very seriously – at least most of the time. So, what are some nutrient-dense healthy choices that will add those extra needed calories?

- Nuts – great source of protein and fat and may protect you from heart attacks. Pine nuts pack the biggest caloric wallop at 673 calories for 3 ounces, but macadamias are no slouch either at 600 calories for 3 ounces.
- Peanuts and Peanut Butter – I know you already knew peanuts are NOT nuts. They are legumes and contain more than 30

essential nutrients and phytonutrients. They also contain Vitamin E, niacin, which helps lower cholesterol, and magnesium, which increases metabolism. 2 tablespoons of this miraculous stuff contains 7 grams of protein and 188 calories.

- Avocados – They're jam packed with antioxidants, vitamins, folate and potassium (60% more than bananas!). They're a great source of unsaturated fat and have been shown to reduce cholesterol when used to replace saturated fats like cheese. One avocado has 300 plus calories.
- Dried Fruit – Dried fruits contain more nutrients, greater fiber content and significantly greater phenol antioxidants as their fresh counterparts. Because it has been dried, its nutrients and calories are very concentrated. Dried fruits include apples, apricots, bananas, blueberries, cherries, grapes, mangos, papayas, peaches, pineapple, dates and figs. A small box of raisins has 129 calories, and cherries weigh in at 160 calories for a mere third of a cup!
- Olive Oil – 1 tablespoon of this golden, green goodness has 120 calories. Use it to cook, on salads, to dip whole grain bread in... This could be the ultimate condiment!
- Protein Shakes, smoothies, shakes and fresh squeezed juices – Celebrate your

need for extra calories and either hit up your local organic juice bar or make your own nutrient dense, calorie laden beverages! Just be sure the ingredients in the Protein Shakes contain high quality undenatured whey protein, that hasn't been exposed to high heat and had its amino acid cellular structure altered. And go light on even the natural sugars.

Fasting for all those hours seems overwhelming. What can I do to make it easier?

The first thing you can do to make intermittent fasting easier is to transition into it at your own pace. Start by fasting for as long as you feel comfortable and build up to the fasting program's recommended hours. If this feels like cheating, start with restricted time fasting, and if at first, even those hours of fasting feel overwhelming build up to their recommendations. This is a life choice; not a diet. Life choices take a lifetime to truly master. Here are some additional tips to help you on your intermittent fasting journey:

- Begin your fast after dinner – Eat your last meal around 7 pm. Go directly to Bed! Wake up at 7 am and BAM! 12 hours of your fast are already over. That's right! Sleep is the beginning faster's best friend!
- Drink Plenty of Water, Tea, Coffee, Sparkling Water, Cold Brewed Teas and

Coffees...Fill that empty stomach with hydrating zero calorie beverages. If you're not overly sensitive to caffeine, the coffee and teas will also give you a lift!

• Don't EVER fast more than two 24-hour periods in one week (this does not, of course count time restricted fasting, as you break that fast for 8 hours each day). Fasting up to two times a week basically cuts up to 30% of your calories. Fasting more than this cuts calories too much and may result in loss of energy and strength and could actually cause boomerang overeating!

How do I coordinate my training schedule to my intermittent fasting schedule?

If you use the fasting and feeding times of your intermittent fasting plan as the boundaries for your training sessions, you will end up with fasted training time that is followed by a replenishing main meal, provided you eat the appropriate foods that complement the workout you've just completed. Here's an example:

Noon: Do workout in fasted state

1 PM: Break 16- hour fast and consume 30 – 50% of daily calories by eating large meal with protein shake

7 PM: Eat balance of calories by eating large dinner

9PM – 1PM Next day: Fast for 16 hours

Please note: This is only an example. While it's important to follow a fasted workout with an ample, replenishing meal, the balance of the day's calories can be eaten at will, as long as the fasted state begins again at 9 pm

Is it ok to drink diet soda when I fast intermittently?

Ummm... Yessss... but why would you want to do that? Sorry about answering a question with a question – but it makes me pause to think that anyone – never mind a health-minded individual, still drinks diet soda. I don't mean to be blunt; but IT'S CHEMICALS, PEOPLE! There. I feel like I've done my duty. The other reason is, there is evidence-based proof that when you drink artificially sweetened beverages, you crave...SUGAR. Not a good thing, and I've got the generation of obese, type two diabetic children to prove it. There are so many great natural alternatives out there – If you need the bubbles, why not try sparkling water or seltzer in at least 50 different flavors – all still coming in at zero calories? Then there's cold brew packs of fruit and spice flavored teas and coffees – delicious as well as warming, soothing hot herbal and caffeinated teas. You can get organic "loaded" and decaf coffee, also in a variety of flavors and from coffee growers around the globe. It's probably the best time in history for zero calorie beverages.

Consider yourself a purist? Consider water – nature's eternal life source! And remember – you are only limited to zero calorie beverages during the fasted state. As you virtuously sip away you can plan ahead for all the delicious juices, lattes and smoothies that await you – in just a matter of hours!

Should I take vitamins when I intermittently fast?

It is more important than ever to take vitamins and supplements when fasting, as you are skipping meals that were helping to supply you with these vital nutrients and it's important that you replace them. The biggest problem with vitamins and fasting is that taking a vitamin pill in a fasted state may result in stomach pain, nausea and diarrhea. To avoid these unpleasant, unsettling effects, try and get your vitamins down while in the fed state. If this is impossible, try taking your vitamins at night so you can sleep through the discomfort.

Alternatively, you might choose vitamins in liquid form, as they are easier to digest while fasting. If you don't normally take vitamins, a basic multivitamin that provides 100% of your daily intake is a great start to ensure you aren't missing out on anything while intermittently fasting.

Why would anyone fast who doesn't want to lose weight?

It may seem odd to someone who is considering intermittently fasting in order to lose weight, for anyone who has their weight under control to change their eating habits or patterns. After all, aren't they already living the dream? Let's not forget about all the other benefits of intermittent fasting:

- Fasting for athletes: Fasting offers a consistent method of fueling and resting the body that works under many of the same principles as training and rest days. It offers them a much more convenient way to ensure that they consume the food they need to train than the other option of eating small meals every 2 or 3 hours, and it allows them to maintain a nutrition routine that provides a lengthier feeding time which can be enjoyed with friends and family.
- Fasting for health benefits: There are people who swear by fasting because they feel it improves their sleep, mental clarity, and helps them control and maintain chronic diseases such as diabetes, cardiovascular disease, multiple sclerosis, fibromyalgia, chronic fatigue syndrome, cancer and the side effects from chemotherapy.
- Fasting for busy people with poor eating habits: People who travel a lot for business often end up feeling less than well most of the time, due to poor eating habits developed as a result of airport restaurants and late-night vending machines. Establishing a consistent intermittent

fasting schedule, including preplanned but convenient and portable food items, allows for much better nutrition, and often fits in well with lengthy travelling times.

- Fasting for financial health and wellness: Which of these two scenarios sounds like a better way to save money? Buying cheap prepared foods like ramen noodles, frozen pizzas and hamburger helper and eating them 24/7 at will, or fasting for 16 hours a day, then eating fresh homemade salads, cooked beans, whole grains and chicken during your eight-hour feeding window? I rest my case.

How should I prepare myself to fast intermittently?

Before embarking upon an intermittent fasting program, it will help to mentally and physically prepare for the challenge ahead. There's definitely a mindset process involved in successful intermittent fasting as well as some practical physical considerations.

- Consult your medical practitioner before beginning ANY new eating program. This is standard boilerplate language, but there's a reason for it – it's a necessary step if you are going to embark on intermittent fasting in an informed, safe manner.

- Make sure you are well-hydrated and avoid salty or sugary foods before you fast.

- Don't stuff yourself the night before you fast. This "last supper" mentality is a rookie mistake that will give you indigestion, a poor night's sleep and an even ruder awakening to your stomach and brain when you follow up the preceding evening's bacchanalia with a fasting period.

- Mentally prepare: Remind yourself several times that you are not going to starve to death – that intermittent fasting is a measurable period of time that you have CHOSEN not to eat within. The first step is fasting. The second is feeding. The third step? Repeat!

- Develop an intermittent fasting mindset: Here's the thing – if you start a fasting period and 5 minutes into it you're thinking, "I'm never going to get through this – I'm already hungry and I can't do this." Guess what? You know the answer. If, however you start a fasting period and 5 minutes into it you're thinking, "I'm feeling strong. I don't eat when I sleep for hours and hours. I know I can do this", chances are, you will in fact succeed. In the words of sociologist William Thomas, "If men define situations as real, they are real in their consequences." Interestingly, this holds equally true for both of the mental scenarios above!

What should I eat to break my intermittent fast?

The basic philosophy behind beginning a feeding after an intermittent fasting period is to eat as if you had never fasted to begin with, or forget about the fasting period and carry on normally. That said, it's always interesting to try and define "normal". Remembering your intentions for intermittently fasting in the first place can be a great help when planning the meal you will break the fast with.

If your intention is to lose weight by fasting intermittently, then you should break your fast with a moderate meal full of nutrient dense, healthy food that fuels your intention without out flooding it with tons of empty calories. If your intention is to support your athletic training regime by fasting intermittently, then you should break your fast, especially after a fasted training, with 30 to 50% of your allotted daily calories, to replenish and fuel your physical activity.

If your intention is to improve your overall health and wellness by intermittently fasting, you should break your fast with clean, organic whole foods that support your intention and have specific nutritional benefits that jive with your specific health challenges. If your intention is to save time and/or money by intermittently fasting, then you should break your fast with a frugal but healthy food selection that has been prepared in a manner that allows you to eat with a minimum of monetary expenditure and/or further fanfare.

Why do I get headaches when I fast and how can I stop them?

Complaints of headaches especially when beginning an intermittent fasting program are quite common. If you are waking with a headache, you may not have hydrated yourself enough the night before. Sleeping with a carafe of water and a glass beside your bed can help remedy this situation. Not drinking enough water is generally one of the biggest culprits of headaches during fasting and water should be imbibed throughout the fasting/feeding process. And remember: we get about 40% of our daily water needs from the food we eat, so it makes perfect sense that you need to replace that water during intermittent fasting periods. Headaches can also be a side effect of the detoxing process that occurs in intermittent fasting and will be especially prevalent in the beginning stages of incorporating the program into your health regime.

Caffeine in the form of black coffee or green tea can be your friend in this case as long as you drink it in moderation and are not hypersensitive to the jittery side effects of caffeinating. A headache during intermittent fasting could also signal a need for more salt, which can be remedied by drinking bouillon or adding more salt to your food during feeding periods. Finally, a headache during intermittent fasting could be signaling low blood sugar, and if they continue despite trying all the tricks and tips above, you should consult your doctor and have your blood sugar tested.

Isn't intermittent fasting just a fancy way of saying I'm starving myself?

In a word, NO! You are voluntarily choosing to refrain from eating for a finite period of time of not more than a total of 48 hours in a seven-day period. Let me bring the actual scientific facts of the process of starvation in to help me convince those of you who still don't believe me...

The Process of Starvation

- **PHASE ONE: After three days,** fatty acids are used by the body as an energy source for muscles, but lower the amount of glucose that travels to the brain. Fatty acids also include a chemical called glycerol that can be used, like glucose as an energy source, but it too, will eventually run out.

- **PHASE TWO can last for up to weeks** at a time. The body mainly uses stored fat for energy. A breakdown occurs in the liver and turns fat into ketones, which are groups of three water-soluble molecules. The brain uses these ketones for energy along with any remaining glucose. At this point the body slows down the breakdown of protein.

- **PHASE THREE:** Fat stores are depleted and the body turns to stored protein for energy, breaking down muscle tissue. The muscle tissue breaks down very quickly. When all sources of protein are gone, cells can no longer function.

- **DEATH BY STARVATION** is usually from cardiac arrest, an infection or other result of tissue breakdown. The body does not have the energy to fight off bacteria and viruses. Generally, it takes **8 to 12 weeks** to starve to death, although there have been cases of people surviving **25 weeks or more**.

Now then... my apologies if this seems a bit brutal, but I think I've graphically shown the difference between intermittent fasting and starvation.

I've heard intermittent fasting isn't safe for women... What are the facts?

Women are more hormonally sensitive than men. Because of this, they may respond more intensely to the challenges of intermittent fasting, and need to consult with a medical professional before starting an intermittent fasting program, especially if they have menstrual and/or fertility issues. Once intermittent fasting has been undertaken, women should also pay special attention to their menstrual cycle, and seek medical guidance if they begin missing periods.

There is a modified or "crescendo" technique of intermittent fasting that will help women who experience hormonal sensitivity. This is a more gradual approach that will help the female body adapt to fasting. Here are the basic rules:

- Fast on 2-3 nonconsecutive days per week
- On fasting days, stick to light workouts such as yoga or light cardio
- Fast for 12-16 hours
- Save strength training for feeding periods or feeding days
- Drink loads of water
- After a few weeks, add another day of fasting and monitor how it goes.

Why can't I have a protein shake when I'm fasting?

Because protein shakes are a MEAL replacement option! Even though they are marketed for their nutrient-density, are packed with protein, are convenient and easily digestible they are, technically FOOD. You can't eat food when you are intermittently fasting – hence you can't drink a protein shake. People get confused about protein shakes – check out diet, fitness, and nutrition and health websites if you don't believe me. I used to shake my head in wonder when I first saw this question asked.

Now I've had a change of heart and have decided to educate rather than ridicule! If you look at the nutrition label on a protein shake you will see that they contain anywhere from 100 to 300 plus calories a shake. If you are on a 5:2 type of intermittent fasting program and you are consuming 500 to 600 calories on your "low" days, feel free to indulge in one or 2 of these shakes if they don't bring you over your total calorie count. If you are on Whole Day Fasting or in the fasting portion of your Time Restricted intermittent fasting cycle don't even think about it!

How can I fast when I'm on vacation?

I indirectly referred to the answer to this question when I was explaining some of the advantages of Whole Day Fasting and 5:2 Intermittent Fasting. Because you are confining your fasting to 2 non-consecutive days of the week, you can automatically end up with a 4-day feeding unit of time. This will help the eating challenges of holidays and vacations in a big way. Another option would be to switch to time restricted intermittent fasting during vacations and holidays, so that there is an 8-hour period during each day for you to eat socially and/or indulge a bit. It might be fun, also to think outside of the traditional food-centric box for a moment, and plan a holiday or vacation that isn't all about overindulging.

Sign everyone up for a half marathon or a day's biking or hiking tour! It's easier to stick to intermittent fasting during festive times if you have company doing it. Finally, giving yourself a week or two break from intermittent fasting doesn't need to be the end of the world. As long as you get back to plan sooner than later, you'll be back in business before you know it and no worse for the break.

Can intermittent fasting really be a long-term weight loss solution?

Honestly, I believe that intermittent fasting is THE solution for long-term weight loss! My reasoning is that because it is NOT a diet, but a lifestyle choice with flexible options, intermittent fasting can be a vital part of the rest of your LIFE. I've already established that this is a sustainable, flexible, balanced, cost-effective timesaving way to incorporate healthy weight loss into your health regime. I've also touted the additional health benefits, including better sleep, mental clarity, increased longevity and preventative protection against a host of chronic diseases caused by poor diet and overindulgence. There is no time limit on intermittent fasting; it will flex and accommodate your health and nutrition needs throughout your weight loss journey and onward through future weight maintenance challenges.

Can I stop fasting once I reach goal weight?

Of course, you can...but WHY would you? If you have taken the time and effort to acclimate yourself to intermittent fasting AND it helped you achieve your personal weight loss goal, why would you go BACK to "diet-think" and stop the program once you reached goal? This type of thinking and finite goal-driven weight loss systems that were devised around this philosophy is precisely WHY people generally don't tend to keep the weight off and worse still, WHY they not only gain back the weight they originally took off, but bounced at the bottom like a trick yoyo and catapulted up to new weight highs!

Think of intermittent fasting programs like this: The constants, or boundaries of these plans are the FED state and the FASTED state of being. These are both natural states for all human beings, and as a matter of fact, human beings are constantly in either one state or another. So why not regulate these states? This is where the variables, or flexibility options come in. By regulating how long you are in the fasted state vs how long you are in the fed state, you can control how long your body ingests and digests food and how long your body rests, burns stored energy sources and detoxes and repairs. You regulate these times, and you can adjust them to your personal needs and goals.

Following an intermittent fasting program that automatically provides you with a consistent, sustainable set of nutritional boundaries, within which you can vary how much and what kinds of food you want to introduce to your body, depending upon and balancing between your needs and desires. In the end, as with so many sustainable platforms, it comes down to balance. Finding and establishing balance are the hard parts of the equation. With the help of intermittent fasting, maintaining this balance becomes manageable and sustainable throughout a lifetime.

Common Fasting Mistakes And How To Avoid Them

At this point I am more than a bit hopeful that you, too are ready to begin your intermittent fasting journey. But, before you start, I've listed some of the mistakes people make while fasting as well as ways you can avoid making them too.

Quitting before you give intermittent fasting a fighting chance:

It's a lifestyle! Yes - it's a challenging transition but the potential rewards are AMAZING! I've read many an account of people who have basically fasted for two and half hours and called it quits. For Pete's sake, everyone can fast for at least 6 hours right out of the box. How do I know that? Because even the worst sleeper (have I mentioned that intermittent fasting can improve your sleep?) has had a "restful" 6 hours of sleep every once in a while. One of the most visceral accounts of this "quitting out of the gate" mentality was a man who journaled about preparing for his first intermittent fast. I read with growing interest, as he parroted back his positive research findings, added up all the potential benefits, and ate his last meal in preparation for the BIG event. He literally wrote about the first couple of hours then stopped.... In the middle of a sentence! It was like, "I'm now twenty minutes into my second hour and I have to say ..." That's all he wrote! I laughed out loud, but

I also felt kind of sad for him. Sad for the missed opportunity. Sad that no one told him to take intermittent fasting at his own pace. Sad that he felt like he had failed again and probably "rewarded" himself by eating everything in the kitchen cupboard.

I'm going to ask you to please give intermittent fasting at least 30 days – one month to try it out and experience the changes it makes. And please don't limit yourself only to pounds lost. Take measurements every week. Journal how your sleep is and how your energy ebbs and flows. Write about your food choices and how you feel about the food you eat after a fasting period. Are you drawn to new and/or different foods than you have been in the past? Has the amount you eat changed? How often are you eating during feeding periods? At the end of the 30 days, put it all together. I think you'll be pleasantly surprised that you did, and I'll be shocked if you're not!

Going whole Hog on your first fast:
There is no humiliation in easing into intermittent fasting. Take advantage of the many different intermittent fasting plans in existence and "date" a couple of them before making a big commitment. You may find that several plans resonate more than others, and want to mix and match plans or create your own hybrid. Just remember the golden rules: No more than two 24-hour period fasts per

week, and no two 24-hour fasts on consecutive days. For time restrictive plans, don't go more than 16 hours each day without feeding for the balance of the 24 hours.

Alternatively, design your own gradual immersion schedule to acclimate yourself to intermittent fasting gracefully. You could accomplish this either by gradually extending the periods you fast or by gradually decreasing the hours you feed. The choice is yours as long as the goal of intermittent fasting remains authentic and the golden rules are adhered to.

Eating as much crappy food as you can!

So, you've been intermittently fasting religiously. You've got the timing down to the second and you never cheat...during the fast. But when it's feeding time...Souie!!! All bets are off and any indulgence is fair game. Okay. Deep breath. Let's have a reality check. Are you really surprised you haven't lost much weight, or you don't feel so great or you're experiencing a lot of gastric distress? It is an amazing fact about human beings: we can take pretty much any "best practice" and warp it right out of recognition! It doesn't matter how good you are at the fasting part if you put bad gas in your tank at the end of the day. Here's a good rule of thumb if you're having a hard time coming to terms with the fact you can't eat like a drunken frat boy and lose weight by fasting intermittently:

Just because you CAN (eat like a lumberjack) doesn't mean you SHOULD.

You sit around and wait for the results...
Basically, especially when you first start intermittently fasting, it's highly advisable to keep your mind and body doing something so you don't sit around obsessing on the fact that you can't eat. Don't clear your schedule for your first fast. Live your life and let it fill you instead of food. Try and schedule activities that aren't about food in any way. Don't tempt yourself by hanging around people who can (and will) eat. Avoid break rooms and snack cabinets at the office. Take a miss on the third birthday party cake-fest this week! Give yourself a break and take a nice long walk. Watch your favorite comfort show on Netflix or give yourself permission to take a well-deserved afternoon nap. You will be amazed, and perhaps a bit startled by how much food there is in western culture; how we idolize it, covet it and include it every time we gather to mark an important event; be it a joyous wedding or a somber funeral. It will give you pause – take that pause to reflect and decide how much you want food in your life.

Going overboard with the "stimulants":
So, caffeine in the form of coffee and tea is totally allowed when you intermittently fast and that's a good thing. But, you know what they say about too

much of a good thing... Remember the whole balance thing so your pleasant morning coffee "euphoria" doesn't turn into a raging case of café nervosa! Too much caffeine will wreak havoc with your stomach and your nervous system. Drink coffee and tea mindfully, always keeping your personal tolerance levels in mind.

Fearing "the hunger":
Learn to recognize and come to terms with casual hunger. Know, with the growing assurance that comes with acclimating yourself to intermittent fasting, that casual hunger is a passing thing. You have the knowledge to understand that short term fasting doesn't cause the body to "devour its own" muscle tissue or cause any other bodily harm. Don't let your mind play games with your intentions.

Overtraining:
While it's true that you might get away with intense workouts on fasting days, why take the chance of overextending or even injuring yourself? It is a simple fact that you will most likely feel better if you give your body a bit of a break on fasting days. Experts recommend taking a miss on long aerobic or cardio workouts on days when you are taking in less fuel. Try a more replenishing session of yoga or stretching instead, to prevent

the discomfort and worry of dizziness or weakness.

Ignoring body temperature changes when fasting:

Some people experience an internal temperature drop when fasting. This is a stress response so respond to it. Dress warmly and don't push yourself in any way that would add additional stressors to your day.

In terms of intermittent fasting MORE does not equal BETTER:

There is a very good, scientific reason why you shouldn't fast more than two full days a week? Simply put, most benefits of intermittent fasting decline at the full day mark. If you find yourself stretching out your fasting periods past the recommended times, you need to rethink things. This would be a good place to consider the difference between fasting and starvation.

In terms of intermittent feeding LESS does not equal MORE:

Be very careful not to start cutting down on your food intake to see if you can lose more weight faster. Intermittent fasting is about moderation and balance between fasting and feeding. Don't tip this beautiful balance by cheating yourself out of the food you need to stay healthy. If you feel like this might be happening, seek medical help immediately!

Don't stalk the clock:

How ironic is it that the very same people who celebrate the freedom and flexibility that intermittent fasting affords them often fall victim to endless and obsessive clock watching during fasting AND feeding periods. If you fall into this category, try and reinforce the flexibility of fasting by deregulating the exact times you eat during your feeding window. Experiment with snacking. Vary your mealtimes and make allowances for social interaction and special events. Be mindful about developing rigidity around eating. And on the fasting side, if you start or end your fasting period a bit from time to time don't let it ruin your day. Remember, with intermittent fasting every day offers the gift of another opportunity to get your health and wellness right!

Forgetting that it's a cohesive system:

Try not to get caught up in the details of either fasting or feeding. Like the "mind-body connection" that alternative health gurus and personal coaches espouse more and more these days, you can't experience the sum total benefits of intermittent fasting if you don't let the two parts of the plan work together in harmony.

Ignoring what your body is trying to tell you:
At the end of the day, intermittent fasting is only going to be good for you if your body accepts it. If you experience any symptoms besides the slight physical discomforts already discussed, you need to stop the fast immediately. This includes, vomiting, fainting, shortness of breath, panic attacks or any unexpected and/or sudden sharp pain. If you don't experience relief soon after stopping the fast, seek immediate medical assistance.

Expecting Miracles:
Don't get me wrong. I think intermittent fasting is the bomb. Why would I be spending all this time and energy writing this book if I wasn't a true believer? BUT: It is not alchemy or wizardry or magic. Done properly and mindfully, intermittent fasting will help you lose or maintain weight, improve many facets of your general health, save you time and money and provide you with a consistent yet flexible nutrition, health and wellness regime. Here's what it won't change:

The negative effect of eating too many of the wrong calories
- o **How big your muscles get if you don't exercise enough or in the correct way**
- o **Junk food into healthy food**

      o **Burning the candle at both ends, by working all day and partying all night**

      o **The fact that you are in the end, "only human", and vulnerable to the ups and downs of this crazy thing we call life!**

A Selection Of Intermittent Fasting "Hacks"

In the interest of giving you the best insight and advice to begin your intermittent fasting journey, I have endeavored to search high and low for helpful tricks and tips to make your experience as productive, user-friendly and successful as possible. Herewith are my findings!

- Start small: There's no such thing as doing too little when it comes to introducing yourself to intermittent fasting. Something as small as shifting your mealtimes by an hour at a time is a step in the right direction
- Keep it simple: Sometimes you fast. Sometimes you feed.
- Focus on flexibility: Rather than getting upset about not eating, focus on the flexibility of intermittent fasting and how much time you are allowed to eat in moderation rather than being on a relentlessly restrictive diet.
- Remember who you are: Be mindful of your likes and dislikes, hopes and fears, personal lines in the sand. In the end, you need to drive the intermittent fasting bus –not the other way around!
- Be prepared for fasting ups and downs. Remember that this is a lifestyle change as well as a change in ingrained habits. Not

easy but not beyond the realm of possibility.

- Remember your goals, but appreciate the process. This is going to take time, so you need to appreciate the journey and not keep asking, "Are we there YET?"
- Learn to listen to your body. Figure out the difference between physical hunger and mental hunger that just might be looking for things beside the instant gratification of food.
- Appreciate the breaks in your routine. Notice how it feels not to have to have to prep a meal or feel obligated to eat at a culturally prescribed time of day.
- Educate yourself about healthy food. Read up on nutrition or go to your local farmer's market and listen to what the experts have to say about their wares.
- Reflect on how much you exercise and why you do it. Listen to your body if it's telling you to stop or urging you to continue an activity.
- Try to be more productive in the morning. Take advantage of when you are fresh from a good night's sleep to accomplish challenging or complicated tasks.
- Don't tell people you are fasting. People can be negative or skeptical about alternative

health practices, no matter how ancient or practical these practices are.

- Indulge sometimes! You are working hard for the greater good of your body. Splurge on dessert every once in a while, to keep yourself in balance. When you eat to live you still have to remember what life is all about!

- Leave your house: If you are living with other people, chances are there are gastronomic temptations behind every door and in every drawer. Give yourself a break and head out for a diverting adventure when you are fasting.

- Make sure your next fast-breaking meal is close at hand. There is no excuse for having to make poor food choices because you don't have healthy food available at the end of a fasting period. It's not like it's a surprise after all!

- Intermittent fasting should simplify your day; not complicate it. If this isn't true, something isn't right. Fix it.

- Fasting begins when you finish your last meal of the feeding period. This detail may seem picky, but it matters.

- Develop a "fasting mindset": project in your mind how the day will go, and prepare yourself for distractions and temptations.

- If it works for you, think about people who have survived shipwrecks, plane crashes, avalanches and other disasters and how they managed to live without food for days and weeks. Your fasting period fears should pale in comparison!
- The key to intermittent fasting is mostly mental. If you can stop listening to other people AND the negative voices in your head full of preconceived notions, old wives' tales and urban myths, you will gain the calm clarity necessary to navigate your fasting journey to healthy feeding!
- The better you are at intermittent fasting the less people will care! It's a fact of life that once the novelty has worn off and there's less chance of failure, other people lose interest in the new and different. Always remember it's about and for you. Not anyone else...
- Make sure your fasting plan fits your lifestyle. Earlier in this book I suggested that certain intermittent fasting plans might be advantageous to people with poor diets who travel a lot. The point is, there are enough IF program options out there to make sure the one you participate in works for your life.
- Eat as healthy a diet as you can afford. Budget the money you save by fasting to

buy the quality food your body deserves when you are feeding.

- Don't use fasting to get out of things. Just like a new baby or a puppy, you will be tempted to use your new fasting routine to get out of social obligations that aren't at the top of your list. Be honest instead of making excuses. Don't cheapen the good things in your life by using them to avoid unpleasantness.

- Be a life-learner: Keep learning all you can about the science behind intermittent fasting. It's miraculous stuff!

- Don't overeat. If there is one thing intermittent fasting should teach you, it's that there will always be another opportunity to eat. Learning delayed gratification eventually teaches us how to quell the needy voices in our hearts.

- Pamper yourself when you are fasting. Pretend you are at an expensive spa and indulge in a long bubble bath. Get a pedicure or massage. Celebrate your healthy body!

- Time your hunger attacks. Generally, hunger pangs will last around 15 minutes. Drink a large glass of water and check the clock.

- Try the "no liquid calories" challenge. Even during feeding times, see how it feels to cut out all liquid that contains calories, including soda, alcohol, juice, and added cream and sugar to your feeding window coffee and tea.

- When you eat, practice eating slowly. This goes hand in hand with overeating. Delayed gratification is a beautiful thing and no one is going to steal your food if you don't gobble it right down.
- Eat nutrient dense foods first. Protein, fruit, vegetables and nuts should get top priority. Save the fats and sugary treats for last. You will end up eating less of them this way.
- Eat when you are hungry during feeding windows. Retrain yourself to really listen for physical hunger and relearn how to take cues from your body and eat with mindfulness and authenticity.
- Change your feeding window. Is there a big food-themed party looming in your future? Fear not! Change that day's feeding window time, and *bon appetit*!
- Save your indulgences for eating with others. When you eat alone, be strict with your intake. This will allow for more flexibility and treats when eating with others.
- Track your results. Tracking is useful in helping you figure out what's working and what's not on your intermittent fasting

adventures, and will help you decide where to make adjustments and modifications.

- Once you have gained confidence, embrace your difference and share your intermittent fasting experience with others. This is still nutritional pioneer territory for a lot of people and as long as you are sure of yourself, you need to share the wealth!

- Stay positive for the long haul. Some say that we are creatures of habit. I would like to amend that statement. I believe we are creatures of bad habit. Making positive changes and sticking to them doesn't always seem to work for humans in the long run. Be on the lookout for old nutritional habits that start poking their tired old noses into new lifestyle choices, when we least expect it or when we are dealing with stress. Understand that just like a person who hasn't smoked in 20 years can light up after hearing bad news, a person who has been faithfully following a solid intermittent fasting regime can very easily pick up a fork, seemingly out of the blue and stick it right into a forgotten junk food indulgence just as fast. When and if this happens, it is more important to recognize the action, figure out what made it happen and then move on, instead of feeling like a failure and eating like one too.

- Here's a great rule to intermittently fast by: You can occasionally eat a "cheat" meal, but you can NEVER cheat by eating during a fasting period!

Establishing New And Healthy Eating Habits

If you google how long it takes to establish a new eating habit, you generally get 21 days as the answer. Where did that number come from? My research says it was determined in the 1950s by a plastic surgeon named Maxwell Maltz who noticed that his patients became accustomed to their new looks in about 21 days. So, there you go! Anyway, in the spirit of intermittent fasting being a lifestyle choice AND a lifelong choice, I say let's not put an arbitrary number on change. Let's make it part of the journey; part of the process.

I think one of the best benefits intermittent fasting offers is the opportunity to establish new and healthy eating habits for the following reasons:

- Intermittent fasting allows you to viscerally experience how the mindful consumption of food affects the fasted body. Each and every day becomes a chance to tweak how and what you fuel your body with, as well as to experience, in real time, how your body reacts to that choice.

- Intermittent fasting gives you the boundaries and support system to learn how to balance food consumption with how efficiently your body utilizes the energy it receives from eating.

- Intermittent doesn't put a time limit on your health, only on your fasting and fed states!
- Intermittent fasting literally GIVES you time, in the form of the fasting state, to reflect on your food choices and make better plans and choices.
- Intermittent fasting has no dependence upon expensive, hard-to-find, and/or exclusive products or ingredients to guarantee its efficacy. You do not need to have any sort of wealth to practice intermittent fasting. In truth, it can be a healthy option for frugal living.
- Intermittent fasting offers a complete system of food management, that can flex to the changes you will experience throughout your life.

Now let's focus on the fuel that energizes intermittent fasting; the food that gives this process viability as well as vitality. Here are some healthy food choices, grouped by the recommended order in which they should be consumed when breaking a fasting period.

- Healthy Protein Options: Seafood; white-meat poultry; milk, cheese and yoghurt; eggs; beans; pork tenderloin; soy; lean beef; meal replacement drinks; cereal or energy bars

- Healthy Fruit Options: Mango; pomegranate; guava; raspberries; oranges; apples
- Healthy Veggie Options: Kale; Brussels sprouts; broccoli; bell pepper; artichokes; spinach
- Healthy Fat Options: Avocados; walnuts; nut and seed butters; olives and olive oil; ground flaxseed; dark chocolate
- Healthy Carb Options: Oatmeal; yams; brown rice; whole grains and whole grain breads and pastas; couscous; quinoa; pumpkin; butternut squash

Eating the first fast-breaking meal in this order ensures that nutrient dense food satisfies and fills you first, instead of sugary, salty, fatty processed food that will stuff you with empty calories and cravings!

Using Your Hand To Portion Your Food

I personally find portioning to be one of the ongoing challenges of my life, basically because I enjoy eating large amounts of food at one sitting! No matter how many times I "educate" myself about portion size and control, I am constantly visually stunned by how small many "normal" single sized portions are. But that's my sad… When I am being mindful, I search out single-serving size items of food as often as I can, sacrificing savings and choice for the comfort of having someone else portion my food appropriately. But there is a better way! You can actually use your hand to figure out units of food! Here's how to do it.

Note: This system was devised to give appropriately sized portions for people who want to lose weight. If you do not need to lose weight but still want a system of measuring your food, you can still use this technique and eat more units per meal.

Protein portions = your palm. One unit of protein should be the size of the portion of your hand between your fingers and your wrist.

Fruits and veggies = the size of two fists. One unit of fruits and/or veggies should be the size of your two clenched fists arranged together at the fingers, ending at the wrists.

Good fats = your thumb. One unit of good fat should be the size of your thumb, from its tip to where it meets your palm.

Healthy carbs = your fist. One unit of healthy carbs should equal the size of one of your clenched fists, ending at the wrist.

This method came from Isagenix, and I think it's pretty foolproof for accuracy and the simple fact that it's impossible to lose your measuring tools! If you arrange your plate of food using this method, and you are counting calories, one meal should come in at a total of 400 to 600 calories. This also gives the non-weight-loss folks a good gauge of their food units and lets everyone keep a "hand"le on portion control. Sorry!

Time and/or Money Saving Meal Preps

Saving money and/or time are major benefits that

can be realized when intermittent fasting. Utilizing the following tricks and tips will also simplify and streamline your intermittent fasting process. Win. Win!

- Buy beans and whole grains in bulk. Beans, oatmeal and other dried whole grains such as brown rice, quinoa and couscous can be an inexpensive source of quality health food when purchased in bulk from supermarkets or large health food stores*

- Cook dried beans and whole grains in a modern pressure cooker. Today's safe, efficient stovetop and electric pressure cookers or instant pots make quick work of cooking dried beans and whole grains like steel cut oatmeal. What used to take an overnight soak and hours of cooking time can now be accomplished in under an hour, giving you enough delicious protein and healthy carb sources for a week's worth of meals in one cooking session. You can use more expensive meat, poultry and fish sources as a condiment to your meals, adding flavor while saving money.

- Pre-portion your food units. Using the hand method explained previously, portion out your food for a week or more at a time and refrigerate or freeze as necessary. I find double zipper sandwich bags to be perfect for this prep.

- Buy 1-pound packages of meat (preferably when on sale). Cut the meat into 4 equal portions, stick each in a sandwich bag, seal and freeze. If you buy 1 pound each of pork, steak, chicken and salmon and prep it this way, you end up with 16 meal portions in 5 minutes!

- Buy local meal services. If cost is not a primary concern, and you are new to the intermittent fasting game, have dietary restrictions, need a wakeup call re: portion size and are low on time or inspiration, find local meal service plans, like Paleo or vegan specialists. The price for 5 meals can be pricey, but the convenience, portion size, nutrition info and culinary prowess and imagination you get can be priceless.

- Set a schedule: work a one-day a week food prep session into your intermittent fasting regime.

- Have the right appliance for the job: keep these time and money-making appliances at the ready for quick and easy feeding meal prep: rice cooker; crock pot; pressure cooker; outdoor grill; Foreman indoor grill; microwave oven.

- Get food wraps, bags and containers at the dollar store. Stock up on all your food prep accessories at these handy discount stores.

- Buy a personal cooler or thermal lunch bag. Buying healthy meals at a restaurant, deli or salad bar can be frustrating and expensive. Bring your food to work and social activities and enjoy the savings as well as guilt free eating!
- Prepped meals are more convenient and definitely better for you than fast food. What's faster than fast food? Prepped meals waiting patiently in your fridge. What's better for you than fast food? Just about anything...
- Spice up your life with seasonings and salts: Nothing puts excitement into basic prepped meals like the addition of fresh or dried herbs, spices and seasonings during the prep and cooking processes. Experimenting with the many differently sourced salts available on the market day will also punch up the flavor of food and add sodium, if you are depleted, to your feeding windows.
- Seeds and nuts are nature's croutons! Sprinkle seeds and nuts over salads, soups and veggies for the texture and taste boost you'd normally rely on croutons and breadcrumbs for.
- If variety ISN'T the spice of your life and you like eating the same meals over and over, prepping large batches of your

favorites, portioning them out, eat at your pleasure and repeat, and repeat....

- Prep, portion and store your meals in mason jars. You can even heat them up in the microwave, once you've removed the lid!
- Check out YouTube videos for inspirational intermittent "feasting" meal preps.

Nutrient Dense Food Swaps

Sometimes it's hard to find nutrient dense foods that can substitute for old, less healthy food standbys. Here are a few innovative swaps to help you in your quest for good health:

- Nut "cheese" spreads for traditional cheese spreads and dips. These are great as sandwich spreads, as a dip with veggies, stirred into pasta or whole grain dishes or used as a dressing on salads. They are a great way to get heart healthy fats into your regime and make a great substitute for processed, fatty, salty cheese spreads.
- Frozen zucchini or peas for some of the frozen fruit in smoothies. Boost the fiber in your healthy smoothie AND decrease sugars.
- Puréed avocado for mayonnaise. Use anytime you would use mayo, including as a sandwich spread, as a binder in tuna, chicken or egg salad, in deviled eggs, and as

a creamy base for dips and salad dressings. You'll be adding fiber, potassium, healthy fat and vitamin E right along with a great flavor boost!

- Dark, leafy greens for iceberg lettuce. Use a variety of these zippy greens in salads, smoothies and wraps (as wraps, too!) for a hearty serving of vitamin K, E, A, C and B, as well as minerals and fiber. Compared to these leafy superheroes, watery, pale iceberg is the "junk food" of the lettuce world.
- Coconut milk for dairy milk. Great for vegans as well as anyone who wants a great source for good fats. Use anywhere and for anything you would use dairy milk, including coffee, in whipped cream, ice-cream and in soups.

Specific 5:2 Minimal Calorie Day Food Choices

If you have chosen the 5:2 intermittent fasting plan and are initially stumped by how to spend your 500 to 600 calories on the two minimal calorie days, here are some options, broken down by meals and snacks.

Breakfast ideas (all under 200 calories):

- Packet of plain organic instant steel cut oatmeal made w/water and topped with 1 tablespoon of raisins
- 1 cup nonfat Greek yoghurt topped with ½ cup thawed, quartered frozen cherries
- 1 hardboiled egg, with ½ apple sliced and 2 teaspoons all-natural peanut butter.

Lunch ideas (all under 200 calories):
- Avocado toast made with 1 slice of whole grain toast, 1/6 of an avocado, mashed with lemon, salt and pepper to taste, sprinkled with a few sunflower seeds
- Skinny burrito in a jar made with ¼ cup salsa, ¼ can drained black beans, ¼ cup reduced fat shredded cheddar cheese and dollop of nonfat Greek yoghurt
- 1 banana with 10 almonds

Dinner ideas (all under 200 calories)
- Chicken lettuce cups made with 2 butter lettuce leaves, ¼ cup shredded chicken breast, matchstick cucumber and carrots, balsamic vinegar, salt, pepper, fresh mint leaves and 1 tablespoon chopped dry roasted peanuts
- Zoodle primavera made with ¼ large zucchini, ¼ of an orange bell pepper, ¼ cup cherry tomatoes, 1 ½ large kale leaves, fresh oregano and basil, 8 ounces cooked down strained tomatoes, 1teaspoon olive

oil, with herbs, spices, salt and pepper to taste.

- Omelet made with 3 egg whites, 1-ounce fat free cheese, 1 thin slice of lean ham, chopped and ½ diced onion.

100 calorie snack options: 1 cup of blueberries; ¾ ounce of sharp cheddar cheese; 1 roasted skinless chicken drumstick, 2 medium kiwis; 2 medium figs; 10 natural blue corn tortilla chips; 1 small baked sweet potato, 2/3 of an ounce of dark chocolate, 25 dry-roasted, unsalted pistachios; 1/3 cup canned red kidney beans; 9 Kalamata olives; 2 cups of watermelon; 1 cup fresh raspberries.

Meal replacement shakes and bars can also help on low calorie 5:2 days. Just be sure to read the nutrition labels for clean, natural ingredients and so you don't underestimate the calorie count. Finally, remember that using the hand portion method will result in a plate of food that will come in at between 400 and 600 calories, so if you are vigilant with the ingredients you could design a main meal for this day, using this method. I end this chapter with what I think is a very apt quote from Dr. Michael Eades, an advocate and participant of intermittent fasting:

"Diets are easy in the contemplation, difficult in the execution. Intermittent fasting is just the opposite – it's difficult in the contemplation, but easy in the execution."

Conclusion: Putting It All Together

As I come to the conclusion of this book, I have a confession to make. Even as I write these words, I am actively experiencing a Whole Day Intermittent Fast! Although I have been an advocate and an active participant of and for intermittent fasting as a life choice and lifestyle for quite some time, researching and writing this book has given me a lot of "food for thought". I hope it has done the same for you.

My intention in writing this book was to immerse the reader in all things relating to intermittent fasting – to offer a primer in this ancient, yet currently trending and ever more popular health and wellness regime. I believe that intermittent fasting is so popular (and has been since the turn of the millennium) because it is grounded in common sense and based upon a physiological cycle that already occurs in each and every one of us: the cycle of the fasted vs the fed state. When we embark on the journey of intermittent fasting we are simply regulating the time that passes between when we feed and when we fast. If you think about western civilization and how plentiful and convenient our food sources have become, paired with how little most of us have to physically expend ourselves to procure it, it only makes sense that we are in sore need of an emergency intervention to regulate the resulting overindulgence and underutilization of and to our physical beings. Enter intermittent fasting!

And yet, as I read personal accounts of what a

positive impact this process has had on countless men and women, I am also struck by how "radical", "extreme" and "out there" intermittent fasting is still perceived by many. Even some of its fiercest advocates and active participants caution in their blogs and articles, not to tell people that you intermittently fast, or, if you insist on being the "strange" one in your crowd and sharing your lifestyle choice, to expect ridicule, derision and skepticism in return for your evangelizing and good intentions. It's important to understand that most of this negative reaction is based upon fear and ignorance. People who don't know better are afraid of fasting. People who haven't been exposed to world religion or medical history or alternative health practices are ignorant when it comes to a health and wellness plan that doesn't docilely float along down the "main stream".

If you purchased this book to learn more about intermittent fasting, I congratulate you for your open mind and forward thinking! As you near the end of this book, I have great hope and anticipation that you have gained a greater understanding about what intermittent fasting is, how it works as a nutrition, health and wellness tool and how it can improve so many elements of your life.

I've covered a lot of material in a relatively brief amount of space, so let's review the highlights. If you have read this book in its entirety and reflected upon its information through the lens of self-improvement, the outcomes should include:

- Understanding the religious, cultural and medical history of this ancient practice
- Understanding the science behind intermittent fasting, including the cellular, hormonal, and systemic impact it can have within the human body
- Comprehending the spectrum of benefits intermittent fasting can offer its active participants, including physical, mental, spiritual, quality of life, behavioral, fiscal, time-saving and personal growth improvements.
- Learning about the flexibility of intermittent fasting through reading about three major types of IF: Whole Day Fasting; 5:2 Intermittent Fasting and Timed Restricted Fasting, but understanding that other methods also exist, as well as hybrids and variations, and that there IS an intermittent fasting program that will resonate with you, whether you follow it completely, or further customize it to your specific needs and desires.
- Acquiring the knowledge that Intermittent Fasting can be successfully utilized to target long-term weight loss as well as life-long maintenance after reaching a healthy weight, through continued fasting as well as physical activity.

- That Intermittent Fasting is also advocated for and utilized by individuals who are not primarily looking for weight loss, but who want to reach and maintain other, equally vital health and wellness goals.
- Recognizing that every individual has many questions about intermittent fasting that need to be answered in a comprehensive manner so that the knowledge gained can be implemented and incorporated into their unique process
- Recognizing that there are mistakes that can be made when embarking on the intermittent fasting journey and becoming aware of these potential pitfalls in a preventative manner
- Concluding that intermittent fasting is NOT a diet or has an expiration date – that it is, instead, a way of healthy living that embraces healthy boundaries as well as the flexibility to grow and change with the natural and inevitable ebb and flow of life itself.

As a writer, I have the great honor of also being a teacher and a guide. But perhaps the biggest benefit I get to continuously reap is the ability writing affords me to be an eternal student of life. I truly enjoyed finally learning what metabolism really meant and being able to figure out my TDEE manually, even though it took me an hour to convert the measurements and see where I had messed up my computation! I will sleep a bit sounder tonight knowing if all the information disappears overnight I can still determine how many calories I need to consume a day to maintain my current weight.

When we are young, we get the opportunity to believe in magic a lot, what with fairy tales, and Disney and Christmas and Harry Potter. When we become adults, the magic is harder to locate. My studies into how the body works, the miraculous ways in which it compensates for disease and repairs itself against the damage we and the environment we exist in inflict upon it, has brought magic back into my life. Then, to be introduced to the process of intermittent fasting, a practice that has been followed since ancient times, when the only proof people could amass for its efficacy was through observation and sheer intuition; a practice that has flourished throughout history, coming in and out of fashion, but never completely disappearing only to reemerge at the turn of a new millennium where it could now be judged by cutting edge scientific knowledge and technology – for this practice to not only survive but endure the tests and research and emerge as the ambassador and benefactor of so many health and wellness benefits.... Well. If that isn't MAGICAL stuff, I surely don't know what is!

So thank you. Thank you for joining me on the intermittent fasting journey. I hope I've convinced you to continue the journey and I wish you luck in your future intermittent fasting ventures. I'm also pleased to announce that I've added a BONUS chapter that includes a variable 10-day introductory fasting plan that incorporates lots of the information I've written about in this book. Enjoy!

*BONUS: 10-Day Introductory Fasting Plan!

The following intermittent fasting plan has been designed to include variations on each day for Whole Day Fasting, 5:2 Intermittent Fasting and Timed Restricted Fasting, to accompany whichever of the three plans you have decided to follow. When planning meals for Whole Day Fasting and Timed Restricted Fasting, as well as the feeding days of 5:2, please employ the Hand portion method I described in this book. If your primary goal is to lose weight, please plate each meal you eat, using one of each of the hand portions. If your goal is NOT to lose weight or you feel that you have cut enough calories during your fasting periods, add additional units of "hand" portioned food as you desire, in half or whole units. Also, where physical activity is indicated, go at your own pace, realistically determining your normal level of activity as sedentary, lightly active, moderately active, heavy exerciser or very heavy exerciser. And, of course confer with a medical professional before embarking on the intermittent fasting journey

Day One (Monday):
- **Whole Day Faster:** Good morning! You are only drinking zero calorie beverages today. Don't forget any vitamins and/prescription medicines, if you didn't take them last night. Stay hydrated and if you decide to

work out today, give yourself a break and take it easy!

- **5:2 Faster:** Good morning! You are only drinking zero calorie beverages today and consuming between 500 and 600 calories. Don't forget any vitamins and/prescription medicines, if you didn't take them last night. Stay hydrated and if you decide to work out today, give yourself a break and take it easy! Try eating five or six 100-calorie snacks, like the ones I listed in the book, interspersed throughout the day and see how that works for you!

- **Timed Restricted Faster**: Good morning! Until you reach hour 16 of your fasting period, you are only drinking zero calorie beverages. Then you will break your fast at hour 16 and eat at will for the next eight-hour fasting period, keeping moderation in mind if weight loss is a goal. If you had an intense workout today, don't forget to consume 30 to 50% of your total daily calories during the first meal you break your fast with. Don't forget any vitamins and/prescription medicines, if you didn't take them last night. Stay hydrated!

Day Two (Tuesday):

- **Whole Day Faster:** Congratulations! You made it through your first whole day fast! How do you feel? Today you are free to eat at will, keeping moderation in mind if weight loss is a goal! Don't forget to "Talk to the Hand" when portioning out your food choices. Feel free to amp up that workout if you wish today. You are in a fed state.

- **5:2 Faster:** Congratulations! You made it through your first 5:2 fasting day! How was it? Today you are free to eat at will, keeping moderation in mind if weight loss is a goal! Don't forget to "Talk to the Hand" when portioning out your food choices. Feel free to amp up that workout if you wish today. You are in a fed state.

- **Timed Restricted Faster:** Congratulations! You made it through your first timed restricted fasting day! How did you do? Until you reach hour 16 of your fasting period, you are only drinking zero calorie beverages. Then you will break your fast at hour 16 and eat at will for the next eight-hour fasting period, keeping moderation in mind if weight loss is a goal. If you have an intense workout today, don't forget to consume 30 to 50% of your total daily calories during the first meal you break your fast with. How's that first meal working for you? If you're having trouble getting all those calories in at one sitting, think about adding a protein shake or eating the meal in shifts! Stay hydrated!

Day Three (Wednesday):
- **Whole Day Faster:** Hey there! It's another day of free eating, keeping moderation in mind if weight loss is a goal! Prep your fasting mindset, for tomorrow is a fasting day. Get a good night's sleep tonight and don't eat too much, too late. Keep feeling the burn exercise wise. You are in a fed state.

- **5:2 Faster:** Hey there! It's another day of free eating, keeping moderation in mind if weight loss is a goal! Prep your fasting mindset for tomorrow is a fasting day. Think about how you want to consume your 500 to 600 calories tomorrow and perhaps, prep for it. Get a good night's sleep tonight and don't eat too much, too late. Keep feeling the burn exercise wise. You are in a fed state.

- **Timed Restricted Faster:** Hello! You're really starting to experience the pattern of timed restricted fasting now. Until you reach hour 16 of your fasting period, you are only drinking zero calorie beverages. Then you will break your fast at hour 16 and eat at will for the next eight-hour fasting period, keeping moderation in mind if weight loss is a goal. If you have an intense workout today, don't forget to consume 30 to 50% of your total daily calories during the first meal you break your fast with. Think about adopting the no liquid calorie rule and only drink zero calorie beverages 24/7. That'll keep you hydrated!

Day Four (Thursday):

- **Whole Day Faster:** Welcome to your second fasting day of the week! You are only drinking zero calorie beverages today. Don't forget any vitamins and/prescription medicines, if you didn't take them last night. Stay hydrated and if you decide to work out today, give yourself a break and take it easy! Why not think about adopting the no liquid calories rule and starting tomorrow, only drink zero calories 24/7? It's up to you!

- **5:2 Faster:** Welcome to your second fasting day of the week! You are only drinking zero calorie beverages today and consuming a total of 500-600 calories. If the snacking worked for you on Monday then go for it. Otherwise try 2 two hundred calorie meals and one snack. Don't forget any vitamins and/prescription medicines, if you didn't take them last night. Stay hydrated and if you decide to work out today, give yourself a break and take it easy! Why not think about adopting the no liquid calories rule and starting tomorrow, only drink zero calories 24/7? It's up to you!

- **Timed Restricted Faster:** Greetings! Until you reach hour 16 of your fasting period, you are only drinking zero calorie beverages. Then you will break your fast at hour 16 and eat at will for the next eight-hour fasting period, keeping moderation in mind if weight loss is a goal. If you have an intense workout today, don't forget to consume 30 to 50% of your total daily calories during the first meal you break your fast with. Today would be a great day to think ahead to weekend plans. Got any brunches or late-night parties looming on the horizon? No sweat. Just shift your 8-hour feeding window to accommodate weekend fun and fast the 16 hours before or after the festivities!

Day Five (Friday):

- **Whole Day Faster:** TGIF and congrats! Look at you with two fasting days under your belt! Today you are free to eat at will, keeping moderation in mind if weight loss is a goal! Plan ahead for weekend fun and try to think where you might go a bit lighter on the food so you can indulge a bit later on. Exercise like you mean it today! You are in a fed state.

- **5:2 Faster:** TGIF and congrats! Look at you with two minimal calorie fasting days under your belt! Today you are free to eat at will, keeping moderation in mind if weight loss is a goal! Plan ahead for weekend fun and try to think where you might go a bit lighter on the food so you can indulge a bit later on. Exercise like you mean it today! You are in a fed state.

- **Timed Restricted Faster:** TGIF and keep on keeping on. Until you reach hour 16 of your fasting period, you are only drinking zero calorie beverages. Then you will break your fast at hour 16 and eat at will for the next eight-hour fasting period, keeping moderation in mind if weight loss is a goal. If you have an intense workout today, don't forget to consume 30 to 50% of your total daily calories during the first meal you break your fast with. Why not try swapping in some mashed avocado for that mayo on your sandwich? So good and so good for you!

Notes and Reflections for ALL Fasters:

Day Six (Saturday):

- **Whole Day Faster:** It's the weekend! Hope you have a fun and active day planned. Today you are free to eat at will, keeping moderation in mind if weight loss is a goal! Pickup football game anyone? You are in a fed state. Why not try swapping in some mashed avocado for that mayo on your sandwich? So good and so good for you!

- **5:2 Faster:** It's the weekend! Hope you have a fun and active day planned. Today you are free to eat at will, keeping moderation in mind if weight loss is a goal! Pickup football game anyone? You are in a fed state. Why not try swapping in some mashed avocado for that mayo on your sandwich? So good and so good for you!

- **Timed Restricted Faster:** It's the weekend. If you've got food-themed plans, go ahead and shift your fasting period and feeding window. Just remember, until you reach hour 16 of your fasting period, you are only drinking zero calorie beverages. Then you will break your fast at hour 16 and eat at will for the next eight-hour fasting period, keeping moderation in mind if weight loss is a goal. If you've made the informed decision to make social, food fun your priority, think about going easier on any workouts. You might need some of those calories at your social gathering!

Day Seven (Sunday):
- **Whole Day Faster:** Sunday already? Don't despair! Today you are free to eat at will, keeping moderation in mind if weight loss is a goal! Go for the Gold, exercise wise. You are in a fed state. Take a moment or two tonight to plan tomorrow's fast. Make sure you've got lots of zero calorie bevs on hand and a to-do list to keep you occupied.

- **5:2 Faster:** Sunday already? Don't despair! Today you are free to eat at will, keeping moderation in mind if weight loss is a goal! Go for the Gold, exercise wise. You are in a fed state. Think about tomorrow's fast and keep tweaking your 500 to 600 calorie menu options if you aren't satisfied or need to mix it up.

- **Timed Restricted Faster:** Sunday already? Did you end up going to that party and watching the sunrise? How's that zero-calorie liquid rule working for you, lol? Ahh well! Today's another day. Until you reach hour 16 of your fasting period, you are only drinking zero calorie beverages. Then you will break your fast at hour 16 and eat at will for the next eight-hour fasting period, keeping moderation in mind if weight loss is a goal. If Today's the day for social, food fun, think about going easier on any workouts. You might need some of those calories at your social gathering!

Day Eight (Monday):
- **Whole Day Faster:** Monday, Monday... You are only drinking zero calorie beverages today. Don't forget any vitamins and/prescription medicines, if you didn't

take them last night. Stay hydrated and if you decide to work out today, give yourself a break and take it easy! Keep busy and enjoy your day

- **5:2 Faster:** Monday, Monday... You are only drinking zero calorie beverages today and eating 500 to 600 calories. How are you spending Today's calorie allowance? If you find yourself on the run, consider a low-calorie protein shake or meal replacement bar! Don't forget any vitamins and/prescription medicines, if you didn't take them last night. Stay hydrated and if you decide to work out today, give yourself a break and take it easy! Keep busy and enjoy your day

- **Timed Restricted Faster:** Monday, Monday... back to the grind. Until you reach hour 16 of your fasting period, you are only drinking zero calorie beverages. Then you will break your fast at hour 16 and eat at will for the next eight-hour fasting period, keeping moderation in mind if weight loss is a goal. If you have an intense workout today, don't forget to consume 30 to 50% of your total daily calories during the first meal you break your fast with. So, what did you think of your first week? Have you lost any weight? Lost any inches? Gained any insight?

Day Nine (Tuesday):
- **Whole Day Faster:** You are rocking these fast days! Today you are free to eat at will, keeping moderation in mind if weight loss is a goal! Workout for all you're worth. You are in a fed state. So, what did you think of your first week? Have you lost any weight? Lost any inches? Gained any insight?

- **5:2 Faster:** You are rocking these fast days! Today you are free to eat at will, keeping moderation in mind if weight loss is a goal! Workout for all you're worth. You are in a fed state. So, what did you think of your first week? Have you lost any weight? Lost any inches? Gained any insight?

- **Timed Restricted Faster:** I don't know about you, but Tuesday's my good news day! Until you reach hour 16 of your fasting period, you are only drinking zero calorie beverages. Then you will break your fast at hour 16 and eat at will for the next eight-hour fasting period, keeping moderation in mind if weight loss is a goal. If you have an intense workout today, don't forget to consume 30 to 50% of your total daily calories during the first meal you break your fast with. What's your favorite protein source? If you've never tried plant-based protein, my advice for you is beans. If you're a beans and greens fan, why not venture into the land of Tofu?

Day Ten (Wednesday):

- **Whole Day Faster:** Time flies when you're on a fast! Today you are free to eat at will, keeping moderation in mind if weight loss is a goal! Keep on truckin'! You are in a fed state. I am so PROUD of you and I hope you are too! Keep referring to this plan if it's worked for you and feel free to continue making it your own.

- **5:2 Faster:** Time flies when you're on a fast! Today you are free to eat at will, keeping moderation in mind if weight loss is a goal! Keep on truckin'! You are in a fed state. I am so PROUD of you and I hope you are too! Keep referring to this plan if it's worked for you and feel free to continue making it your own.

-

- **Timed Restricted Faster:** Time flies when you're on a fast! Until you reach hour 16 of your fasting period, you are only drinking zero calorie beverages. Then you will break your fast at hour 16 and eat at will for the next eight-hour fasting period, keeping moderation in mind if weight loss is a goal. If you have an intense workout today, don't forget to consume 30 to 50% of your total daily calories during the first meal you break your fast with. I am so PROUD of you and I hope you are too! Keep referring to this plan if it's worked for you and feel free to continue making it your own.

RECIPES

DELICIOUS EGG AND VEGGIE MUFFINS

SERVES 4 PREPARATION TIME 15 MINUTES
COOKING TIME 25 MINUTES

INGREDIENTS
**6 organic eggs
1 tsp. olive oil
¼ cup chopped onion
2 cups chopped spinach
½ cup diced tomato
½ tsp. pepper
¼ tsp. salt
1 ¼ tbsp. coconut milk**

INSTRUCTIONS

1. Preheat oven to 350°F then prepare 8 muffin cups. Coat the muffin cups with cooking spray then set aside.

2. Preheat a medium skillet then pour olive oil into it.

3. Stir in chopped onion and sauté until translucent and aromatic.

4. Add chopped spinach to the skillet then cook until the spinach is wilted but still green. Remove the skillet from heat.

5. Crack the eggs then place in a bowl.

6. Season the eggs with salt and pepper then mix well.

7. Add diced tomato, coconut milk, and sautéed spinach to the beaten eggs then stir until combined.

8. Pour the mixture into the prepared muffin cups then bake for approximately 20 minutes or until the eggs are set.

9. Remove from the oven then let them cool for a few minutes.

10. Take the egg muffins out from the cups then arrange on a serving dish.

11. Serve and enjoy.

NUTRITION PER SERVING
CALORIES 126 PROTEIN 9.2 FIBER 0.9 SUGARS 2

FAT 9

TIP

For a healthier choice, use organic eggs for this recipe.
For variation, you can add some other vegetables such as mushrooms, carrots, broccoli, or kale.

CHEESY HAM BURRITOS

SERVES 4 PREPARATION TIME 10 MINUTES
COOKING TIME 10 MINUTES

INGREDIENTS
8 slices ham
4 organic eggs
2 tsp. minced garlic
¼ tsp. salt
¼ tsp. pepper
3 tsp. butter
¾ cup grated cheese
½ cup chopped broccoli

INSTRUCTIONS

1. Crack the eggs then place in a bowl.

2. Season the eggs with salt and pepper then whisk to combine.

3. Preheat a skillet over medium heat then add 1 teaspoon of butter to the skillet.

4. Stir in minced garlic then sauté until lightly golden and aromatic.

5. Add chopped broccoli to the skillet then cook until wilted.

6. Pour egg mixture into the skillet then let it sit for about 10 seconds.

7. Using a wooden spatula, stir the egg mixture; lift, and fold the eggs until scrambled. Remove from heat then set aside.

8. Place a slice of ham on a flat surface then add a tablespoon of the egg and broccoli mixture then top with cheese. Roll the ham and prick with a toothpaste. Repeat with the remaining ingredients.

9. Preheat a pan over low heat.

10. Brush the rolled ham with the remaining butter then place in the pan.

11. Sauté until the ham is crispy then place on a serving dish.

12. Repeat with the remaining ham and filling then serve immediately.

13. Enjoy.

NUTRITION PER SERVING

CALORIES 271 PROTEIN 20.6 FIBER 1.1 SUGARS
0.7 FAT 19.1

TIP

Mozzarella cheese is a great choice for its
meltability. However, if you don't have mozzarella
cheese in your kitchen, cheddar cheese is fine.
Avoid overcooking the egg. A soft and runny
texture for the scrambled egg is best for this
recipe.

STUFFED AVOCADO WITH BLACK PEPPER CHICKEN

SERVES 4 PREPARATION TIME 10 MINUTES COOKING TIME 10 MINUTES

INGREDIENTS
2 ripe avocados
½ lb. cooked chicken
1 tbsp. chopped onion
¼ tsp. salt
½ tsp. black pepper
2 tbsp. water
1 tsp. olive oil

INSTRUCTIONS

1. Preheat a skillet then pour olive oil into it.

2. Stir in chopped onion then sauté until wilted and aromatic.

3. Cut the cooked chicken into very small dice then pour water over the chicken.

4. Season with salt and pepper then cook until the water is completely absorbed. Remove from heat then set aside.

5. Preheat an oven to 250°F.

6. Cut the avocados into halves then fill with the chicken filling.

7. Bake the avocado for about 10 minutes then transfer to a serving dish.

8. Enjoy.

NUTRITION PER SERVING

CALORIES 227 PROTEIN 4 FIBER 6.9 SUGARS 0.6
FAT 21

TIP
If you don't have cooked chicken, you can substitute it with tuna, eggs, or any kinds of vegetables, as you desire.

SOFT CAULIFLOWER CAKES WITH SHRIMP

SERVES 4 PREPARATION TIME 20 MINUTES
COOKING TIME 20 MINUTES

INGREDIENTS
3 cups cauliflower florets
¼ cup grated carrot
2 tbsp. chopped leek
¼ cup fresh shrimp
2 tsp. minced garlic
2 organic eggs
½ cup grated cheese
¼ tsp. salt
¼ tsp. pepper

INSTRUCTIONS

1. Peel the shrimp then place in a food processor.

2. Add cauliflower florets and minced garlic to the food processor then pulse until the cauliflower florets becoming crumbles.

3. Transfer the cauliflower florets crumble to a mixing bowl then add grated carrot and

chopped leek to bowl. Mix well then set aside.

4. Crack the eggs then place in a bowl.

5. Season with salt and pepper then whisk until incorporated.

6. Pour the egg mixture into the cauliflower florets then mix well.

7. Preheat an oven to 250°F then coat a baking pan with cooking spray.

8. Pour the cauliflower florets mixture into the prepared baking pan then spread evenly.

9. Sprinkle grated cheese on top then bake for about 20 minutes or until it is set.

10. Remove from the oven and let it cool for a few minutes.

11. Remove from baking pan then cut into medium squares.

12. Serve and enjoy warm.

NUTRITION PER SERVING

CALORIES 134 PROTEIN 12.5 FIBER 2.2 SUGARS
2.5 FAT 7.2

TIP
You can also bake this dish in disposable
aluminium muffin tins. Though it will be more
expensive, for sure, it will also be more practical as
you don't have to wash the baking pan.
Besides, if you bake this dish in small cups, you can
enjoy it as an on-the-go breakfast.

SAVORY ALMOND CAKES

SERVES 4 PREPARATION TIME 12 MINUTES
COOKING TIME 32 MINUTES

INGREDIENTS
¾ cup almond flour
3 organic eggs
¼ cup almond milk
2-¼ tbsp. almond butter

INSTRUCTIONS

1. Preheat an oven to 375°F then line a square baking pan with parchment paper. Set aside.

2. Melt the butter then set aside.

3. Crack the eggs then place in a bowl.

4. Using an electric smoker, whisk the eggs until fluffy.

5. Add almond flour to the eggs then mix well.

6. Pour almond milk and almond butter into the mixture then stir well.

7. Pour the batter into the prepared baking pan then spread evenly.

8. Bake for approximately 30 minutes or until you can prick with a toothpick and it comes out clean.

9. Remove from the oven then place on a cooling rack.

10. Once it is cool, take the cake out of the pan then cut into squares.

11. Arrange on a serving dish then enjoy.

NUTRITION PER SERVING

CALORIES 161 PROTEIN 7.3 FIBER 1.7 SUGARS 1.3 FAT 14

TIP

If you like, cheese can be added to this recipe. Cut the cheese into small cubes then add to the batter. The cake will taste so cheesy! You can also sprinkle grated cheese on top.

SPECIAL NUTTY PORRIDGE

SERVES 4 PREPARATION TIME 5 MINUTES
COOKING TIME 10 MINUTES

INGREDIENTS

2 ¼ cups unsweetened almond milk
½ cup almond butter
2 tbsp. almond oil
¼ cup chia seeds
¼ cup toasted chopped pecans
¼ cup toasted chopped walnuts
¼ cup roasted sliced almond
1 tsp. cinnamon

INSTRUCTIONS

1. Pour almond milk into a pan then bring to a simmer.

2. Stir in chia seeds, pecans, walnuts, and sliced almonds, then stir well. Remove from heat.

3. Quickly add almond butter and almond oil to the pan then stir well.

4. Transfer to a serving dish then sprinkle cinnamon on top.

5. Serve and enjoy.

NUTRITION PER SERVING

CALORIES 263 PROTEIN 5.7 FIBER 5.9 SUGARS 1
FAT 24.4

TIP
This nutty porridge can be enjoyed hot or cold.
If you like, you may add cloves and nutmeg to
enhance the aroma.

SOFT COCONUT WAFFLES

SERVES 4 PREPARATION TIME 5 MINUTES
COOKING TIME 15 MINUTES

INGREDIENTS
**4 organic eggs
3 tbsp. coconut flour
2 tbsp. coconut yogurt
3 tbsp. butter**

INSTRUCTIONS

1. Melt the butter then let it cool.

2. Crack the organic eggs then place the egg yolks and egg whites in separate bowls.

3. Using an electric mixer, whisk the egg whites until fluffy then set aside.

4. Whisk the egg yolk then combine with the coconut flour.

5. Add butter to the mixing bowl then stir until combined.

6. Next pour the coconut yogurt over the batter then mix well.

7. Preheat a waffle maker then cook the waffles according to the instruction manual.

8. Once cooked, remove from the waffle maker then repeat with the remaining ingredients.

9. Serve and enjoy

NUTRITION PER SERVING

CALORIES 186 PROTEIN 7.2 FIBER 3.8 SUGARS 1.3 FAT 14.6

TIP
Enjoying these waffles with granola is not only delicious but also beneficial. As you know, granola contains lots of good nutrients for the body.

SCRAMBLED EGGS WITH AVOCADO

SERVES 4 PREPARATION TIME 5 MINUTES
COOKING TIME 15 MINUTES

INGREDIENTS
**6 organic eggs
1 tbsp. olive oil
½ tsp. black pepper
2 tbsp. chopped leek
1 ripe avocado**

INSTRUCTIONS

1. Peel the avocado then discard the pit.

2. Cut the avocado into cubes then set aside.

3. Crack the eggs then place in a bowl.

4. Season with black pepper then stir until incorporated.

5. Preheat a saucepan over medium heat then pour olive oil into the saucepan.

6. Add the egg to the saucepan then let it sit for about 15 seconds.

7. Stir and fold the eggs until scrambled.

8. Add chopped celery and avocado cubes to the saucepan then mix well.

9. Transfer to a serving dish then enjoy.

NUTRITION PER SERVING

CALORIES 229 PROTEIN 9.3 FIBER 3.5 SUGARS 0.9 FAT 19.9

TIP

Avocado in this recipe is a variable ingredient. You may substitute it with tomato, spinach, bacon, or other ingredients, as you desire.

CHICKEN CARROT FRITTATA

SERVES 4 PREPARATION TIME 10 MINUTES
COOKING TIME 25 MINUTES

INGREDIENTS

5 organic eggs
½ tsp. olive oil
½ cup chopped onion
½ cup grated carrot
¼ cup coconut milk
½ tsp. pepper

INSTRUCTIONS

1. Preheat an oven to 250°F.

2. Crack the eggs then place in a bowl. Whisk until incorporated.

3. Preheat a pan over medium heat then pour olive oil into it.

4. Stir in chopped onion then sauté until wilted and aromatic.

5. Add carrot to the skillet then season with pepper.

6. Pour coconut milk over the carrot then bring to a simmer.

7. Next, turn the stove off then pour the egg into the pan. Spread evenly.

8. Bake the carrot frittata for approximately 25 minutes or until the eggs are set.

9. Once it is done, remove from the oven then serve.

10. Enjoy warm.

NUTRITION PER SERVING

CALORIES 125 PROTEIN 7.6 FIBER 1.1 SUGARS 2.2 FAT 9.1

TIP
This carrot frittata is good with homemade sugar-free tomato sauce.

BAKED PUMPKIN WITH CINNAMON

SERVES 4 PREPARATION TIME 10 MINUTES
COOKING TIME 55 MINUTES

INGREDIENTS
1 ½ tbsp. olive oil
3 cups pumpkin cubes
1 tsp. cinnamon
½ tsp. black pepper

INSTRUCTIONS

1. Preheat an oven to 325°F then prepare a baking sheet.

2. Place pumpkin cubes on a sheet of aluminium foil then splash olive oil over the pumpkin.

3. Sprinkle with cinnamon and pepper then wrap the pumpkin with aluminium foil.

4. Bake the pumpkin for about 40 minutes then remove from the oven.

5. Unwrap the pumpkin then bake again for about 15 minutes.

6. Once the pumpkin is done, remove it from the oven,

7. Transfer the baked pumpkin to a serving dish.

8. Serve and enjoy.

NUTRITION PER SERVING

CALORIES 71 PROTEIN 1 FIBER 1 SUGARS 1.2 FAT 5.4

CHEWY ALMOND BAGELS

SERVES 4 PREPARATION TIME 15 MINUTES
COOKING TIME 15 MINUTES

INGREDIENTS
**1 cup almond flour
1-¾ cups grated Mozzarella cheese
2 tbsp. softened cream cheese
2 organic eggs
2 tbsp. sesame seeds**

INSTRUCTIONS

1. Preheat an oven to 400°F and line a baking sheet or baking pan with parchment paper.

2. Place the almond flour in a mixing bowl then add eggs and softened cream cheese to the bowl.

3. Knead the almond and eggs until becoming dough then add grated Mozzarella cheese to the dough. Knead until just combined.

4. Divide the dough into 4 then shape each part into bagel form.

5. Arrange the bagels on the prepared or lined baking sheet then sprinkle sesame seeds on top.

6. Bake the bagels for about 15 minutes or until the bagels are lightly golden with a firm texture.

7. Take the bagels out from the oven then place on a cooling rack. Let them cool.

8. Arrange on a serving dish then serve.

9. Enjoy.

NUTRITION PER SERVING

CALORIES 135 PROTEIN 7.5 FIBER 1.3 SUGARS 0.4 FAT 10.9

TIP

At the beginning, the dough will be a bit sticky. However, keep kneading until becoming a dough form.
If you have an electric mixer with kneading function, you can use it for a better and faster result.

CINNAMON SOUFFLE DELIGHT

SERVES 4 PREPARATION TIME 15 MINUTES
COOKING TIME 25 MINUTES

INGREDIENTS

1 tbsp. almond butter
½ cup almond flour
½ tsp. cinnamon
1 cup unsweetened almond yogurt
½ cup cheese cubes
6 organic eggs
¼ cup roasted chopped almond

INSTRUCTIONS

1. Preheat an oven to 350°F then brush 4 medium soufflé cups with melted butter.

2. Crack the eggs then place in a mixing bowl.

3. Using an electric mixer whisk the eggs until smooth and fluffy.

4. Add almond flour and cinnamon to the eggs then whisk until incorporated.

5. Next, pour almond yogurt into the mixture then mix well.

6. Add cheese cubes to the batter.

7. Using a spoon, stir the batter until just combined.

8. Divide the batter into 4 prepared cups then sprinkle chopped almonds on top.

9. Bake the soufflés for about 25 minutes or until the soufflés are set and the top is lightly golden.

10. Remove from the oven then place on a cooling rack.

11. Serve and enjoy warm.

NUTRITION PER SERVING

CALORIES 135 PROTEIN 7.5 FIBER 1.3 SUGARS 0.4 FAT 10.9

TIP

It is highly recommended that you cut the cheese into cubes and not grate it. The cubed cheese will give a more intense taste than grated cheese.

PUMPKIN EGG CASSEROLE

SERVES 4 PREPARATION TIME 12 MINUTES
COOKING TIME 20 MINUTES

INGREDIENTS
**3 cups pumpkin cubes
3 organic eggs
2 tsp. cinnamon
¾ cup unsweetened almond milk
2 tbsp. almond flour**

INSTRUCTIONS

1. Preheat an oven to 250°F then coat a medium casserole dish with cooking spray.

2. Spread the pumpkin cubes in the prepared casserole dish then set aside.

3. Crack the eggs then place in a bowl.

4. Combine coconut flour with coconut milk then pour the mixture into the eggs. Whisk to combine.

5. Pour the egg mixture over the pumpkin then sprinkle cinnamon on top.

6. Bake the pumpkin casserole for about 20 minutes or until the casserole is set.

7. Once it is done, take the casserole out of the oven then let it cool for a few minutes.

8. Serve and enjoy.

NUTRITION PER SERVING

CALORIES 85 PROTEIN 5.5 FIBER 1.3 SUGARS 1.3 FAT 4.5

ORIGINAL COCONUT PANCAKES

SERVES 4 PREPARATION TIME 8 MINUTES
COOKING TIME 10 MINUTES

INGREDIENTS
2 organic eggs
2 tbsp. flax seeds
½ cup coconut flour
½ cup coconut milk
1 tsp. olive oil

INSTRUCTIONS

1. Combine all ingredients in a bowl then whisk until smooth and incorporated.

2. Preheat a saucepan over medium heat then brush with olive oil.

3. Pour about 2 tablespoons of batter into the saucepan then cook for about 2 minutes.

4. Flip the pancake then cook again for another 2 minutes or until both sides of the pancake are lightly golden.

5. Repeat with the remaining batter then arrange on a serving dish.

6. Serve and enjoy.

NUTRITION PER SERVING

CALORIES 136 PROTEIN 4.4 FIBER 2.2 SUGARS
1.4 FAT 11.9

TIP
Top the pancakes with fresh fruits according to
your desire.

WARM SPINACH SMOOTHIE

SERVES 4 PREPARATION TIME 2 MINUTES
COOKING TIME 6 MINUTES

INGREDIENTS

2 cups unsweetened almond milk
2 cups chopped spinach
2 medium carrots
2 tbsp. lemon juice
2 tsp. ginger

INSTRUCTIONS

1. Peel the carrots then cut into thick slices.

2. Place the carrots in a blender then add the remaining ingredients to the blender. Process until smooth.

3. Divide the smoothie into 4 serving glasses then serve.

4. Enjoy.

CALORIES 41 PROTEIN 1.3 FIBER 1.7 SUGARS 1.8
FAT 1.9

TIP
This smoothie is also great consumed cold. Make it
at the night before and store it in the refrigerator.

SAVORY VEGETABLE PANCAKES

SERVES 4 PREPARATION TIME 5 MINUTES
COOKING TIME 15 MINUTES

INGREDIENTS

¼ cup coconut flour
½ tsp. pepper
1 organic egg
2 tbsp. coconut milk
½ cup grated carrot
½ cup zucchini
1 cup chopped spinach
½ cup chopped onion
1 ½ tbsp. olive oil

INSTRUCTIONS

1. Combine coconut flour with pepper, egg, and coconut milk. Stir well.

2. Add carrot, zucchini, spinach, and onion then mix well.

3. Preheat a saucepan over medium heat then brush the pan with olive oil.

4. Drop about two tablespoons of batter to make the pancake. Repeat with the remaining ingredients.

5. Arrange the pancakes on a serving dish then serve immediately.

NUTRITION PER SERVING

CALORIES 98 PROTEIN 2.4 FIBER 1.5 SUGARS 2 FAT 8.3

LOW CARB CHEESE SANDWICH

SERVES 4 PREPARATION TIME 6 MINUTES
COOKING TIME 12 MINUTES

INGREDIENTS
8 organic eggs
½ cup mashed avocado
4 slices bacon
4 slices cheddar cheese

INSTRUCTIONS

1. Preheat a steamer then coat 8 small round baking pans with cooking spray.

2. Crack the eggs and place each egg in each baking pan.

3. Arrange the pan in the steamer then steam until the eggs are set— like making steamed sunny side up eggs.

4. Remove the baking pan from the steamer then take the steamed sunny side up eggs out of the baking pan.

5. Arrange 4 steamed eggs on a flat surface then spread mashed avocado over each egg.

6. Layer with bacon and cheese then top with the remaining steamed eggs.

7. Arrange on a serving dish then serve.

8. Enjoy.

NUTRITION PER SERVING

CALORIES 287 PROTEIN 18.6 FIBER 2 SUGARS 0.9 FAT 22.5

TIP
Make sure that you use ripe avocados for this recipe. Unripe avocados have a hard texture and bitter taste.

ZUCCHINI CUPCAKES WITH TASTY BACON

SERVES 4 PREPARATION TIME 20 MINUTES
COOKING TIME 25 MINUTES

INGREDIENTS
2 medium zucchinis
4 slices bacon
1 cup almond flour
¼ cup chopped onion
¼ tsp. salt
½ tsp. pepper
4 organic eggs
3 tbsp. water

INSTRUCTIONS

1. Preheat an oven to 250°F then coat 8 muffin cups with cooking spray.

2. Peel the zucchini then discard the seeds.

3. Shred the zucchini then set aside.

4. Cut the bacon into very small dice then place in the same bowl with grated zucchini.

5. Add chopped onion to the same bowl then mix well.

6. Crack the eggs then place in a separate bowl.

7. Season with salt and pepper then using an electric mixer whisk until fluffy.

8. Pour water into the beaten egg then add almond flour into it. Whisk until incorporated.

9. Add the zucchini mixture to the egg mixture and using a wooden spatula stir well.

10. Pour the mixture into the prepared muffin cups then bake for 20 minutes or until the tops of the cupcakes are lightly golden.

NUTRITION PER SERVING

CALORIES 138 PROTEIN 8.9 FIBER 2.2 SUGARS 2.6 FAT 9.6

TIP

This on-the-go breakfast can be prepared in advance so you can save time in the morning. Store this dish in a container with a lid in the refrigerator. When you want to consume, microwave on medium heat for 30 seconds then enjoy.

SALMON PLATTER

SERVES 4 PREPARATION TIME 7 MINUTES
COOKING TIME 10 MINUTES

INGREDIENTS
8 organic eggs
2 radishes
1 ripe avocado
1 tsp. olive oil
¼ tsp. salt
¼ tsp. pepper
1 cup sliced salmon

INSTRUCTIONS

1. Crack an egg then into a bowl.

2. Pour water into a saucepan then bring to a simmer.

3. Once it is simmering, gently slip the egg into the water.

4. Poach the egg until set but still soft. Repeat with the remaining eggs, cooking only one egg at a time.

5. Next, preheat a saucepan over medium heat then pour olive oil into it.

6. Once it is hot, stir in salmon fillet then season with salt and pepper.

7. Sauté until salmon is just cooked then remove from heat.

8. Divide the salmon into 4 serving dishes then add two poached eggs to each dish.

9. Peel the avocado and discard the pit. Cut the avocado flesh into small dice.

10. Place diced avocado and sliced radish on each dish then serve the salmon platter.

11. Enjoy.

NUTRITION PER SERVING

CALORIES 329 PROTEIN 22.1 FIBER 3.4 SUGARS 1 FAT 25.2

LEMON SOUFFLE WITH STRAWBERRY TOPPING

SERVES 4 PREPARATION TIME 15 MINUTES
COOKING TIME 20 MINUTES

INGREDIENTS
12 egg yolks
12 egg whites
1 ½ tsp. lemon zest
3 tbsp. lemon juice
¼ cup coconut flour
3 tsp. coconut oil
TOPPING:
1 cup fresh strawberries
½ cup water
2 tbsp. lemon juice

INSTRUCTIONS

1. First, make the topping.

2. Place fresh strawberries in a pan then pour water and lemon juice over the strawberries.

3. Bring to a simmer while stirring occasionally.

4. Remove from heat and let sit for a few minutes until thickened.

5. Meanwhile, preheat an oven to 250°F then coat a medium baking dish with cooking spray. Set aside.

6. Place egg yolks together with lemon zest, coconut flour, and coconut oil in a bowl. Whisk until incorporated.

7. In a separate bowl, place egg whites and lemon juice then whisk until foamy.

8. Stir in the egg whites to egg yolk mixture then mix until combined.

9. Pour the egg mixture into the prepared baking dish then spread evenly.

10. Drizzle strawberry topping on top then bake the casserole for approximately 20 minutes.

11. Once it is done, remove from the oven then let cool.

12. Serve and enjoy.

NUTRITION PER SERVING

CALORIES 262 PROTEIN 19.4 FIBER 1.1 SUGARS
3.2 FAT 17.5

TIP

Strawberry can be substituted with blueberry,
cranberry, raspberry, or a mix of these fruits.
Choose ripe berries, so you can enjoy the natural
sweetness.

VEGETABLE WAFFLES

SERVES 4 PREPARATION TIME 15 MINUTES
COOKING TIME 15 MINUTES

INGREDIENTS

1 cup grated carrot
4 organic eggs
¼ cup almond flour
¼ tsp. black pepper
2 tbsp. grated cheese

INSTRUCTIONS

1. Crack the eggs then combine with almond flour.

2. Season with black pepper then whisk until smooth.

3. Add grated cheese and grated carrot to the flour mixture then mix until combined.

4. Preheat a waffle maker then cook the waffles according to the machine's instructions.

5. Arrange the waffles on a serving dish then enjoy.

NUTRITION PER SERVING
CALORIES 129 PROTEIN 8.2 FIBER 1.5 SUGARS 2
FAT 9

TIP
If almond flour is too expensive, consider coconut
flour as a cheaper option.

SOFT CINNAMON PANCAKE

SERVES 4 PREPARATION TIME 4 MINUTES
COOKING TIME 15 MINUTES

INGREDIENTS
½ cup softened cream cheese
8 organic eggs
½ cup almond yogurt
1 tsp. cinnamon

INSTRUCTIONS

1. Crack the eggs then place in a mixing bowl.

2. Add softened cream cheese to the bowl then using an electric mixer whisk until smooth and fluffy.

3. Add almond yogurt and cinnamon to the batter then mix well.

4. Preheat a pan over medium heat then coat the pan with cooking spray.

5. Drop about two tablespoons of batter then make the pancake. Repeat with the remaining ingredients.

6. Arrange the pancakes on a serving dish then serve immediately.

NUTRITION PER SERVING

CALORIES 248 PROTEIN 13.8 FIBER 0.8 SUGARS 1 FAT 20.1

TIP

If you like fresh fruit, you can add diced fresh strawberry or blueberry to the batter.

QUICK TOMATO FRITTATA

SERVES 4 PREPARATION TIME 10 MINUTES
COOKING TIME 15 MINUTES

INGREDIENTS
10 organic eggs
1 cup chopped onion
¾ cup crumbled feta cheese
1 cup cherry tomatoes
1 tbsp. butter
2 tbsp. chopped parsley
¼ tsp. salt
½ tsp. black pepper

INSTRUCTIONS

1. Preheat oven to 200°F.

2. Crack the eggs then season with salt and pepper. Whisk until incorporated.

3. Preheat a pan over medium heat then add butter to the pan.

4. Once the butter is melted, stir in chopped onion then sauté until aromatic. Remove from heat.

5. Pour the eggs into the pan then spread evenly.

6. Top the frittata with crumbled feta cheese and halved cherry tomatoes then bake for approximately 10 minutes or until the frittata is set.

7. Remove from heat and let it cool.

8. Serve and enjoy.

NUTRITION PER SERVING

CALORIES 278 PROTEIN 18.7 FIBER 1.3 SUGARS 4.4 FAT 20

TIP

Add some other ingredients that you like to this frittata. Mushrooms, sausage, ground beef, or vegetables are all great choices.

CREAMY ASPARAGUS QUICHE

SERVES 4 PREPARATION TIME 15 MINUTES
COOKING TIME 60 MINUTES

INGREDIENTS
CRUST:
½ cup almond flour
1 organic egg white
1 tbsp. butter
FILLING:
3 organic eggs
1 organic egg yolk
2 tbsp. cooked ground beef
½ cup almond milk
2 tbsp. grated cheese
½ cup chopped asparagus
¼ tsp. salt
¼ tsp. pepper
¼ tsp. nutmeg

INSTRUCTIONS

1. Preheat oven to 375°F then coat a medium pie pan with cooking spray.

2. Combine almond flour with egg white and butter then mix until it becomes a sticky dough.

3. Put the dough into the prepared pie pan then press on the bottom and up the side of the pan.

4. Bake the crust for about 10 minutes then take it out of the oven. Set aside.

5. Crack the eggs then place in a bowl. Season with salt, nutmeg, and pepper.

6. Add egg yolk to the bowl then whisk all until fluffy.

7. Pour almond milk into the eggs then stir well.

8. Sprinkle ground beef and asparagus over the crust then pour in the egg and almond milk mixture.

9. Sprinkle grated cheese on top then bake for about 30 minutes.

10. Once it is done, remove from the oven then place on a cooling rack.

11. Take the quiche out of the pan then cut into wedges.

12. Serve and enjoy.

NUTRITION PER SERVING

CALORIES 308 PROTEIN 19.6 FIBER 1.5 SUGARS
1.8 FAT 24.4

TIP

Do not over bake the quiche to keep the filling soft
and to avoid the crust burning. Once the filling is
set, remove from the oven.

BEEF AND CAULIFLOWER IN PAN WITH AVOCADO

SERVES 4 PREPARATION TIME 10 MINUTES
COOKING TIME 30 MINUTES

INGREDIENTS
**2 tbsp. butter
1 cup chopped onion
1 cup ground beef
¼ tsp. salt
½ tsp. black pepper
1 cup cauliflower florets
5 organic eggs
1 ripe avocado**

INSTRUCTIONS

1. Preheat oven to 250°F then coat a casserole dish with cooking spray. Set aside.

2. Preheat a skillet over medium heat then add butter to the skillet.

3. Once the butter is melted, stir in chopped onion then sauté until wilted and aromatic.

4. Add ground beef to the skillet then season with salt and pepper. Cook for a few minutes until the beef is no longer pink.

5. Stir cauliflower florets into skillet then cook until just wilted. Remove from heat.

6. Transfer the cooked beef and cauliflower florets to the prepared casserole dish then spread evenly.

7. Crack the eggs then drop on the beef mixture—you don't have to beat the eggs -- just let them drop, sunny side up onto the beef mixture.

8. Peel and cut the avocado into halves then discard the pit.

9. Cut avocado into cubes then sprinkle on top.

10. Bake the casserole for about 30 minutes then remove from the oven.

11. Let it cool for a few minutes then serve.

12. Enjoy.

NUTRITION PER SERVING

CALORIES 333 PROTEIN 13.3 FIBER 4.7 SUGARS
2.5 FAT 28.1

REFRESHING COCONUT PORRIDGE WITH BLUEBERRIES

SERVES 4 PREPARATION TIME 10 MINUTES
COOKING TIME 10 MINUTES

INGREDIENTS
2 tbsp. butter
½ cup coconut flour
1 cup coconut milk
1 cup fresh blueberries
½ cup sliced roasted almonds

INSTRUCTIONS

1. Combine coconut flour and coconut milk in a pan then stir until incorporated. Bring to a simmer.

2. Next, stir butter into the pan then cook until the butter is melted.

3. Transfer the porridge to a serving dish then sprinkle chopped blueberries and roasted almonds on top.

4. Serve and enjoy.

NUTRITION PER SERVING

CALORIES 210 PROTEIN 3.6 FIBER 3.1 SUGARS
5.1 FAT 19.1

CAULIFLOWER RICE IN BELL PEPPER BOWLS

SERVES 4 PREPARATION TIME 15 MINUTES
COOKING TIME 40 MINUTES

INGREDIENTS
**4 big bell peppers
2 tbsp. olive oil
½ cup ground beef
¼ tsp. pepper
½ cup chopped onion
2 cups cauliflower florets**

INSTRUCTIONS

1. Microwave the cauliflower florets for a few minutes until crispy.

2. Place the crispy cauliflower in a food processor then process until the cauliflower florets becoming crumbles.

3. Preheat a large skillet over medium heat then pour olive oil into it.

4. Stir in chopped onion and ground beef then sauté until the onion is aromatic and the ground beef is no longer pink.

5. Add cauliflower florets to the skillet then season with pepper. Remove from heat.

6. Preheat oven to 250°F then line a baking sheet with aluminium foil.

7. Cut the bell peppers on top, hollow out then fill each bell pepper with the cooked beef and cauliflower rice.

8. Bake the bell peppers for 30 minutes then remove from the oven.

9. Arrange on a serving dish then enjoy.

NUTRITION PER SERVING

CALORIES 181 PROTEIN 10.1 FIBER 3.3 SUGARS 5.5 FAT 12.2

Natasha Brown

BUTTERY EGG SALAD

SERVES 4 PREPARATION TIME 7 MINUTES
COOKING TIME 5 MINUTES

INGREDIENTS
8 organic eggs
½ cup butter
½ tsp. pepper

INSTRUCTIONS

1. Place egg in a pot then pour water over to cover. Bring to boil.

2. Once it is boiled, reduce the heat then cook the eggs for about 10 minutes.

3. Strain the eggs then let them cool.

4. Peel the eggs then using a spoon chop them.

5. Add butter to the eggs then season with pepper. Mix well.

6. Serve and enjoy.

NUTRITION PER SERVING

CALORIES 330 PROTEIN 11.3 FIBER 0.1 SUGARS
0.7 FAT 31.8

TIP

Place the boiled eggs under cold running water to
help them cool faster.

CHICKEN LETTUCE TACO

SERVES 4 PREPARATION TIME 12 MINUTES
COOKING TIME 15 MINUTES

INGREDIENTS

1 lb. boneless chicken breast
½ cup chopped onion
2 tbsp. butter
2 tbsp. coconut aminos
¼ cup water
1 handful fresh lettuce

INSTRUCTIONS

1. Preheat a skillet (use medium heat) then add butter to the skillet.

2. Once the butter is melted, stir in chopped onion then sauté until wilted and aromatic.

3. Cut the chicken into small cubes then add to the skillet.

4. Pour water over the chicken then cook until the water is completely absorbed.

5. Season with coconut aminos then stir well. Remove from heat.

6. Place fresh lettuce on a flat surface then top each lettuce with cooked chicken.

7. Fold the lettuce then place on a serving dish.

8. Serve and enjoy.

NUTRITION PER SERVING

CALORIES 281 PROTEIN 33.4 FIBER 0.6 SUGARS 0.8 FAT 14.2

TIP

This is a practical lunch that you can eat during busy days. Cook the chicken in double portions then microwave whenever you need.

MIXED CHICKEN VEGETABLE SOUP

SERVES 4 PREPARATION TIME 15 MINUTES
COOKING TIME 18 MINUTES

INGREDIENTS
**3 cups low sodium chicken broth
1 tsp. pepper
1 tsp. minced garlic
½ tsp. nutmeg
1 cup chopped chicken
½ cup chopped carrot
¼ cup mushrooms
2 tbsp. chopped leek
½ cup broccoli florets**

INSTRUCTIONS

1. Place chicken, carrot, and mushrooms in a pot.

2. Pour low sodium chicken broth into the pot then season with minced garlic, pepper, and nutmeg. Bring to boil.

3. Once it is boiled, reduce the heat then cook until the chicken is tender.

4. Bring to boil again then stir in chopped leek and broccoli florets.

5. Once it is done, transfer to a soup bowl then serve warm.

6. Enjoy.

NUTRITION PER SERVING

CALORIES 330 PROTEIN 11.3 FIBER 0.1 SUGARS 0.7 FAT 31.8

TIP

This soup is best eaten fresh. Do not reheat the soup because the vegetables will be overcooked and tasteless.

AVOCADO TUNA SALAD

SERVES 4 PREPARATION TIME 5 MINUTES
COOKING TIME 10 MINUTES

INGREDIENTS

4 ripe avocados
¼ tsp. pepper
2 tbsp. butter
2 tbsp. lemon juice
1 tbsp. chopped parsley

INSTRUCTIONS

1. Peel the avocados and discard the pits.

2. Cut the avocados into cubes then set aside.

3. Splash lemon juice over the tuna then let it sit for about 2 minutes.

4. Next, preheat a skillet then add butter to the skillet.

5. Once the butter is melted, stir in tuna chunks then season with pepper.

6. Using a wooden spatula, stir the tuna until completely cooked then add avocado cubes

to the skillet. Stir until just combined then remove from heat.

7. Transfer to a serving dish then sprinkle chopped parsley on top.

8. Serve and enjoy.

NUTRITION PER SERVING

CALORIES 131 PROTEIN 6.2 FIBER 3.1 SUGARS 0.2 FAT 11.1

TIP

Besides tuna, you can also use salmon, and shrimp for this recipe.
For a healthy twist can add vegetables to this dish.

SAVORY SAUTEED MUSHROOMS

SERVES 4 PREPARATION TIME 5 MINUTES
COOKING TIME 10 MINUTES

INGREDIENTS
4 cups chopped mushrooms
2 tsp. olive oil
3 tsp. minced garlic
½ tsp. black pepper
2 tsp. red chilli flakes
1 tbsp. sesame seeds
¼ cup chopped tomato
1 cup low sodium chicken broth

INSTRUCTIONS

1. Preheat a skillet over medium heat then pour olive oil into the skillet.

2. Stir in minced garlic then sauté until lightly golden and aromatic.

3. Add chopped mushrooms to the skillet then season with pepper and chilli flakes.

4. Pour low sodium chicken broth over the mushrooms then cook until the broth reduces by half.

5. Stir in chopped tomato then mix well.

6. Transfer to a serving dish then sprinkle sesame seeds on top.

7. Serve and enjoy.

NUTRITION PER SERVING

CALORIES 58 PROTEIN 3.4 FIBER 1.3 SUGARS 1.6 FAT 3.7

TIP

You can try various mushrooms for this recipe. White mushrooms, oyster mushrooms, Portobello, and shiitake are all good in this recipe.

EGGS IN A CAVE

SERVES 4 PREPARATION TIME 15 MINUTES
COOKING TIME 25 MINUTES

INGREDIENTS
**4 boiled eggs
1 organic egg
2 cups ground beef
¼ tsp. salt
½ tsp. pepper
½ tsp. nutmeg
2 tbsp. coconut flour**

INSTRUCTIONS

1. Peel the boiled eggs then set aside.

2. Preheat a steamer over medium heat.

3. Season the beef with salt, pepper, and nutmeg then mix well.

4. Add egg and coconut flour to the beef mixture then stir to combine.

5. Cover each boiled egg with beef mixture then wrap each in aluminium foil.

6. Place the wrapped eggs in the steamer then steam for about 25 minutes.

7. Take the wrapped eggs out of the steamer then let them cool.

8. When the eggs are cool, unwrap the eggs then cut into halves.

9. Arrange on a serving dish then serve.

10. Enjoy.

NUTRITION PER SERVING

CALORIES 225 PROTEIN 20.5 FIBER 1.4 SUGARS 0.8 FAT 14.3

TIP

You can substitute the beef with chicken, lamb, or fish, as you desire. However, you must add more flour to the mixture because those kinds of meat are less firm than beef.
For a smaller size, use boiled quail eggs for the filling.

MIXED VEGETABLES IN TURMERIC GRAVY

SERVES 4 PREPARATION TIME 8 MINUTES
COOKING TIME 18 MINUTES

INGREDIENTS
1 cup chopped cabbage
½ cup chopped carrot
½ cup chopped green beans
1 tsp. sliced garlic
2 tsp. sliced shallot
½ tsp. coriander
½ tsp. pepper
½ tsp. turmeric
1 lemon grass
1 bay leaf
1 tsp. olive oil
1 cup water
1 cup coconut milk

INSTRUCTIONS

1. Preheat a medium skillet then pour olive oil into the skillet.

2. Stir in sliced garlic and shallot then sauté until brown and aromatic.

3. Add cabbage, carrot, and green beans to the skillet then sauté until wilted.

4. Season the vegetables with coriander; pepper, turmeric, lemon grass, and bay leaf then pour water over the vegetables. Bring to boil.

5. Once it is boiling, pour coconut milk into the skillet then bring to a simmer.

6. Transfer to a serving dish then enjoy warm.

NUTRITION PER SERVING

CALORIES 168 PROTEIN 2.1 FIBER 2.8 SUGARS 3.5 FAT 15.6

CHICKEN MEATBALLS IN TOMATO SAUCE

SERVES 4 PREPARATION TIME 14 MINUTES
COOKING TIME 25 MINUTES

INGREDIENTS
1 lb. ground chicken
2 organic eggs
4 cloves garlic
SAUCE:
1 cup diced tomato
½ cup tomato puree
½ cup low sodium chicken broth
¼ tsp. salt
½ tsp. pepper
½ tsp. nutmeg

INSTRUCTIONS

1. Pour about a quart of water into a pot then bring to boil.

2. Meanwhile, combine ground chicken with eggs and garlic then mix well.

3. Shape the mixture into small balls then set aside.

4. Once the water is boiled, stir in the meatballs and cook until the meatballs are floating.

5. While waiting for the meatballs, pour diced tomato, tomato puree, and chicken broth in a saucepan.

6. Season with salt, pepper, and nutmeg then bring to a simmer.

7. Stir occasionally then remove from heat. Set aside.

8. Once the meatballs are floating, strain the meatballs and place on a serving dish.

9. Drizzle the tomato sauce over the meatballs then serve.

10. Enjoy.

NUTRITION PER SERVING

CALORIES 275 PROTEIN 37 FIBER 1.3 SUGARS 3
FAT 10.9

TIP
If you like, add lemon juice to the sauce. It will give

an extra brightness to the tomato sauce.

All information is intended only to help you cooperate with your doctor, in your efforts toward desirable weight levels and health. Only your doctor can determine what is right for you. In addition to regular check ups and medical supervision, from your doctor, before starting any other weight loss program, you should consult with your personal physician.

FNº

Presented by French Number Publishing
French Number Publishing is an independent
publishing house headquartered in Paris, France
with offices in North America, Europe, and Asia.
FNº is committed to connect the most promising
writers to readers from all around the world.
Together we aim to explore the most challenging
issues on a large variety of topics that are of
interest to the modern society.

FNº

Made in the USA
Monee, IL
08 January 2021